LABORATORY DIAGNOSIS IN NEONATAL CALF AND PIG DIARRHOEA

CURRENT TOPICS IN VETERINARY MEDICINE AND ANIMAL SCIENCE

VOLUME 13

LABORATORY DIAGNOSIS IN NEONATAL CALF AND PIG DIARRHOEA

Series ISBN: 90-247-2429-5

LABORATORY DIAGNOSIS IN NEONATAL CALF AND PIG DIARRHOEA

Proceedings of a Workshop on Diagnostic Techniques for Enteropathogenic
Agents Associated with Neonatal Diarrhoea in Calves and Pigs, held at the
Central Veterinary Institute, Department of Virology, Lelystad, The
Netherlands, June 3-5, 1980

Sponsored by the Commission of the European Communities,
Directorate-General for Agriculture,
Coordination of Agricultural Research

Edited by

P.W. de Leeuw

Centraal Diergeneeskundig Instituut,
Lelystad, The Netherlands

and
P.A.M. Guinée

Rijksinstituut voor de Volksgezondheid,
Bilthoven, The Netherlands

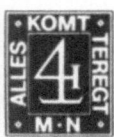

MARTINUS NIJHOFF PUBLISHERS
THE HAGUE / BOSTON / LONDON

for

THE COMMISSION OF THE EUROPEAN COMMUNITIES

Distributors

for the United States and Canada
Kluwer Boston, Inc.
190 Old Derby Street
Hingham, MA 02043
USA

for all other countries
Kluwer Academic Publishers Group
Distribution Center
P.O. Box 322
3300 AH Dordrecht
The Netherlands

ISBN-13: 978-94-009-8330-4   e-ISBN-13:978-94-009-8328-1
DOI: 10.1007/978-94-009-8328-1

Publication arranged by
Commission of the European Communities,
Directorate-General Information Market and Innovation, Luxembourg

EUR 6899

LEGAL NOTICE

Neither the Commission of the European Communities nor any person acting on behalf of the Commission is responsible for the use which might be made of the following information.

CONTENTS

ENTERIC VIRUSES

Preface

In recent years several "new" infectious agents have been
associated with neonatal diarrhoea in both calves and pigs.
Furthermore, important additional information has become
available as regards enterotoxigenic <u>Escherichia coli</u> infections in both species. Although still much has to be learned,
it is likely that in many field cases differnt agents act in
concert. Therefore an integrated approach to the problem
of neonatal diarrhoea appears to be necessary, particularly
in the field research. Such an approach requires a series of
diagnostic techniques.
The purpose of this meeting was to bring together a limited
number of scientists that are actively involved in neonatal
diarrhoea research, in order to discuss present knowledge
and to produce proceedings containing review articles, new
developments and laboratory manuals of relevant diagnostic
techniques.

This publication constitutes a collection of scientific papers and laboratory manuals on diagnostic techniques for enteropathogenic agents in neonatal diarrhoea in calves and pigs, presented and discussed during a workshop in the EEC Programme of Coordination of Agricultural Research on Protection of the Young Animal against Perinatal Diseases, held at the Central Veterinary Institute, Department of Virology, Lelystad, the Netherlands, June 3-5, 1980.

VIRAL AGENTS ASSOCIATED WITH NEONATAL DIARRHOEA AND THEIR DETECTION BY ELECTRON MICROSCOPY

M.S. McNulty, W.L. Curran and J.B. McFerran

Veterinary Research Laboratories, Stormont, Belfast,

BT4 3SD, N. Ireland

ABSTRACT

Simple techniques for diagnosis of enteric viral infections by direct electron microscopy of faeces are described. For best results, some degree of purification and/or concentration of faecal material is necessary. This can be adequately achieved by differential centrifugation. A number of viruses have been observed in the faeces of the domestic animal species and man. These include rotaviruses, coronaviruses, astroviruses, caliciviruses, adenoviruses, parvoviruses and enterovirus-like particles. Mixed infections with combinations of these viruses are extremely common. Caution should be exercised in interpretation of results. Detection of one of the above viruses in the faeces of an animal with diarrhoea does not necessarily indicate etiological significance.

INTRODUCTION

Within the last decade a number of previously unknown enteric viruses have been discovered. Most of these viruses cannot be isolated in cell cultures using conventional techniques, but occur in sufficient numbers in infected faeces to allow them to be detected directly by electron microscopy (EM). In this paper, methods for the direct examination of faecal material by EM are described and results obtained with this technique are reviewed.

MATERIALS AND METHODS

Direct EM examination of faeces

Method A. Make an approximately 15% suspension of crude faeces in 1% ammonium acetate or distilled water. Apply to a grid for a few minutes and stain.

Method B. Dilute faecal material approximately 1:5 to a final volume of about 15 ml in phosphate-buffered saline (PBS). Centrifuge at 3 000 g for 30 min to remove bacteria and gross debris. Collect the resulting supernatant and centrifuge at 91 000 g for 1 h. Resuspend the pellet in a few drops of 1% ammonium acetate or distilled water and examine.

Method C. To about 15 ml of a 15-20% suspension of faeces add an equal volume of the fluorocarbon, Arcton 113 (ICI Ltd, Runcorn, Cheshire, England). Mix thoroughly to form an emulsion. Separate the aqueous and Arcton layers by centrifugation at 3 000 g for 15 min. Remove the upper aqueous layer, ultracentrifuge as described in Method B and examine the pellet.

Immune electron microscopy of faeces

Prepare a clarified faecal suspension as described in Methods B or C above. Add an equal volume of serum diluted with PBS. Either a specific antiserum or pooled sera obtained from adult animals of the same species as the specimens under test may be used. If the titre of the serum is unknown, test it at several dilutions e.g. 1:50, 1:250 and 1:1 000, and subsequently use the dilution which gives the best clumping. Incubate the serum-virus mixture for 2 h at $37^{o}C$ or overnight at $4^{o}C$. Centrifuge at 10 000 g for 30 min and examine the pellet.

Grids and staining

Carbon-coated 400 mesh grids are used routinely at Stormont. Specimens are stained for about 1 min with methylamine tungstate (EMscope Laboratories Ltd, Ashford, Kent, England) or 4% sodium phosphotungstate, pH 6.5.

General considerations

Usually it is necessary to prepare only one grid from each specimen unless they are obviously unsatisfactory. Normally at least 5 or 6 good squares of a 400 mesh grid should be examined before a negative result is reported. At a working magnification of about 40 000 x, this will take about 10 min.

It is advisable to photograph virus-like particles of uncertain identity, as some viruses are difficult to identify unequivocally on the screen. This is particularly important for inexperienced operators, as it allows their results to be checked.

RESULTS

In our experience, it is easier to find virus particles in the contents of the large intestine, caecum and rectum than in small intestinal contents. Consequently the former are the specimens of choice from a dead animal. Sometimes, particularly in the case of young pigs or broiler chickens, it may be difficult to identify animals with diarrhoea or to obtain a sample of faeces from them. In this case it is best to scrape obviously diarrhoeic material off the floor. Animals should be sampled as soon as possible after the onset of diarrhoea as virus titres tend to be highest at this time. Material should be sent to the laboratory in clean, screw-topped, secure containers. No diluent is necessary for EM examination. Many veterinary practitioners submit material collected on cotton wool swabs. These are unsatisfactory for several reasons. They often contain insufficient material and usually yield inferior preparations. Also if submitted dry, virus isolation attempts are likely to be unsuccessful. It is advisable to ask practitioners to submit samples large enough to permit further investigation if new or unusual viruses are found e.g. 10 ml from a calf, 5 ml from a pig.

It should be remembered that EM is not a sensitive technique. Virus at a concentration of 10^5 particles/ml is just at the borderline of detection (Flewett, 1978). Fortunately, however, most of the enteric viruses are excreted in vast numbers in the faeces, 10^{10} rotavirus particles/ml is not uncommon. Method A is very simple and was first described by Middleton et al. (1977), who used it to detect rotaviruses, adenoviruses and a variety of small round viruses in human faeces. We have found it useful for screening bovine faeces for rotavirus and coronavirus. It is not as satisfactory for pig and avian faeces. Pig faeces appear to contain a lot more non-viral contaminating material than bovine faeces and enteric viruses tend to be present in lower numbers in avian faeces than mammalian faeces (McNulty et al., 1979a). For faeces from these species, some degree of purification and/or concentration is necessary. Method B is normally suitable for this purpose. However, if faeces contain a lot of lipid and difficulty is encountered in clarifying suspensions, fluorocarbon extraction as described in Method C may be used.

Small round viruses (calicis, astros etc) are best demonstrated following pelleting, which facilitates observation of groups of particles. Clumping may also be achieved by immune EM. However, it is necessary to use the antiserum at the correct dilution. If antibody is present in too high a concentration, the surface structure of the virus particles will be obscured. Either specific antisera or pooled adult sera may be used for immune EM. Pooled adult sera possess antibodies against a wide range of micro-organisms, so that as general diagnostic reagents they are more useful than hyperimmune sera. Furthermore they have the added advantage of ready availability.

Table 1 lists the viruses which have been detected in the faeces of

4

the domestic animal species and man by direct EM. It is hardly surprising
that the greatest variety of viruses has been recognised in calves and
humans, as these have been the most intensively studied species.

TABLE 1 - VIRUSES DETECTABLE IN FAECES BY DIRECT ELECTRON MICROSCOPY

	Calf	Pig	Lamb	Foal	Dog	Cat	Turkey	Fowl	Human
Rotavirus	+[1]	+[2]	+[3]	+[4]	+[5]	+[6]	+[7]	+[7]	+[8]
Coronavirus	+[9]	+[10,11]	+[12]	+[13]	+[14,30]	+[15]	+[16]		+[17,18]
Astrovirus	+[19]		+[20]				+[21]		+[22]
Calicivirus	+[19]								+[23]
Parvovirus					+[24]				?[25]
Adenovirus									+[26]
Enterovirus-like	+[27]	+[28]			+[5]		+[7]	+[7]	+[29]

1   Mebus et al. (1969)
2   Rodger et al. (1975)
3   Snodgrass et al. (1976)
4   Flewett et al. (1975)
5   Eugster and Sidwa (1979)
6   Snodgrass et al. (1979)
7   McNulty et al. (1979a)
8   Flewett et al. (1973)
9   Stair et al. (1972)
10 Saif et al. (1977)
11 Pensaert and de Bouck (1978)
12 Tzipori et al. (1978)
13 Bass and Sharpee (1975)
14 Appel et al. (1978)
15 Hoshino and Scott (1980)
16 Ritchie et al. (1973)
17 Mathan et al. (1975)
18 Caul et al. (1975)
19 Woode and Bridger (1978)
20 Snodgrass and Gray (1977)
21 McNulty et al. (1980)
22 Madeley and Cosgrove (1975)
23 Madeley and Cosgrove (1976)
24 Eugster and Nairn (1977)
25 Kapikian et al. (1972)
26 Flewett et al. (1975)
27 McNulty et al. (1976)
28 McNulty, unpublished
29 Middleton et al. (1977)
30 Schnagl and Holmes (1978)

Rotaviruses.   Next to bacteriophages, these are the most commonly
encountered viruses in faeces. Regardless of the species of origin, all
rotaviruses are morphologically indistinguishable (Woode et al., 1976;
McNulty et al., 1979b). Intact particles are about 70 nm in diameter.
They have been described as reovirus-like, but can be distinguished from
reoviruses by virtue of their more clearly defined outer edge (Fig. 1.).

Furthermore, reoviruses are very rarely detected in faeces by direct EM, and are never present in the same vast numbers as rotaviruses. The outer shell of rotaviruses may be lost to produce particles which resemble orbiviruses and which are about 10 nm smaller than intact virions.

Coronaviruses. In recent years, there have been many reports of the detection of coronavirus-like particles in the faeces of animals and man, both with and without diarrhoea (Table 1). Some of these particles are morphologically different from classical coronaviruses, as exemplified by avian infectious bronchitis virus, most notably with respect to the surface projections. Caul and Egglestone (1979) have therefore suggested that there may be two subgroups of coronaviruses, one group with the classical petal-shaped projections and the other possessing projections consisting of thin stalks which terminate in spherical or teardrop-like knobs (Figs. 2, 3). However it is by no means certain that all of these coronavirus-like particles are indeed viruses, let alone pathogens.

Of the agents unequivocally shown to be coronaviruses, direct EM of faeces is a useful diagnostic procedure for bovine and canine enteric coronaviruses. The best characterised pig enteric coronavirus is transmissable gastroenteritis (TGE) virus. However, although TGE virus has been demonstrated in the faeces of experimentally infected pigs by immune EM (Saif et al., 1977), virus isolation and/or immunofluorescence are more commonly used for diagnosis (Pensaert and Debouck, 1978; Bohl, 1979). Recently, Pensaert and Debouck (1978) have isolated a new coronavirus from pigs in Belgium with an epizootic diarrhoea similar to TGE. This virus has not yet been isolated in cell cultures but can be detected in faeces by direct EM. Chasey and Cartwright (1978) described a coronavirus-like agent in the faeces of pigs in Britain with epidemic diarrhoea. However, demonstration of this agent by direct EM of faeces is unreliable. Neither TGE nor epidemic diarrhoea are present in Northern Ireland.

Difficulty in recognising coronaviruses will be encountered when partial or complete loss of the main morphological feature i.e. the corona of surface projections, has occurred. It should be remembered that the corona of some coronaviruses is very fragile and may be destroyed by freezing and thawing and/or prolonged storage.

Astroviruses. These are spherical viruses about 28 nm in diameter. Their main distinguishing feature is a star-shaped surface configuration. This can be clearly seen on only about 10% of the particles and may be either a

5- or 6-pointed star which occupies most of the surface of the particle
(Fig. 4). The surface detail may be difficult to recognise on the screen,
underlining the necessity to photograph particles of uncertain identity.
Astroviruses have been detected in only a few animal species (Table 1).
Caliciviruses. Caliciviruses have a well developed star- or lattice-shaped
surface configuration. However, unlike astroviruses, only 6-pointed stars
are present. Furthermore, the calicivirus star has a central hollow
whereas the centre of the astrovirus star is never filled with stain.
Caliciviruses are slightly bigger (31 nm) than astroviruses and have a less
well defined outer edge, with a scalloped as opposed to a circular outline
(Fig. 5). The distinguishing features of caliciviruses and astroviruses
have recently been described in detail by Madeley (1979). Enteric
caliciviruses were first detected in the faeces of children with diarrhoea
by Madeley and Cosgrove (1976). Calicivirus-like agents have also been
isolated from calves (Woode and Bridger, 1978). These have a similar
degree of pathogenicity for gnotobiotic calves as rotaviruses (J.C. Bridger,
personal communication).

Parvoviruses. At present, direct EM is useful for diagnosing parvoviral
enteritis only in dogs. This condition has assumed major importance all
over the world during the last 2 or 3 years. Often the virus is present in
sufficient numbers in the faeces of affected dogs to be detected easily by
Method A (Fig. 6). Parvovirus infections can cause enteritis and diarrhoea
in calves, but virus isolation is the recommended diagnostic method in this
case (Storz and Leary, 1979). A number of human 'parvovirus-like' agents
similar to and including the Norwalk agent have been described (Holmes,
1979). These do not occur in large quantities in the faeces and immune EM
is usually necessary to allow them to be detected (Holmes, 1979). It is
possible that these agents are not, in fact, parvoviruses. They are
slightly larger (26-30 nm) than parvoviruses (18-26 nm) and have not yet
been characterised biochemically.

Adenoviruses. Adenoviruses are sometimes found in very large numbers in
the faeces of humans with diarrhoea. Normally these viruses cannot be
isolated and grown in cell cultures (Flewett et al., 1975; Middleton
et al., 1977). As far as we are aware no truly analagous situation has
been described in animals. Adenoviruses are occasionally encountered in
very small numbers in avian faeces, but these are probably the same viruses
which can be readily isolated in cell cultures (McNulty et al., 1979a).

Enterovirus-like particles.   Small round virus-like particles about 28 nm
in diameter and without any obvious surface structure have been reported in
the faeces of several animal species (Fig. 7, Table 1).   These have not been
isolated in cell cultures and their significance is unknown.

Other virus-like particles in faeces.   Middleton et al. (1977) have
described 30 nm, double-shelled, spherical virus-like particles in the
faeces of children with gastroenteritis and diarrhoea.   These particles
have been called 'mini-reovirus', but at this stage their true nature is
unknown.   One suggestion is that they may be caliciviruses (Holmes, 1979).
The fringed particles about 100 nm in diameter which Mebus et al. (1978)
described in association with villous epithelial cell syncitia and diarrhoea
in calves are not sufficiently distinctive morphologically to permit
reliable diagnosis by direct EM.   Similar particles are regularly
encountered in the faeces of all the domestic species, both from normal
animals and those with diarrhoea.   For the same reasons, BVD/mucosal disease
cannot be diagnosed with certainty by direct EM.

It is important to appreciate that mixed infections with combinations
of the above viruses are extremely common e.g. rotavirus and coronavirus in
calves, rotavirus and enterovirus-like particles in pigs and parvovirus and
coronavirus in dogs.   It is therefore essential to examine each grid
thoroughly and not to stop as soon as the first virus is recognised.

DISCUSSION

It is obvious that direct EM examination of faeces is a potent tool in
diagnosis of enteric viral infections.   As most of the enteric viruses cannot be routinely isolated in cell cultures, it is the only catch-all system
presently available for diagnosis.   It permits very rapid diagnosis for
important specimens and has the important advantage that mixed infections
can be easily recognised.   On the debit side, the basic equipment is
expensive both to buy and to maintain.   The number of specimens which can
be processed by EM is very much lower than that possible using techniques
such as ELISA.   Another limitation is the insensitivity of the technique –
about 10^6 virus particles/ml are required for consistent detection.
Furthermore, as discussed above, some viruses may be difficult to recognise.
However, it is likely that most of the blank spaces in Table 1 will be
filled in during the next few years, and direct EM is probably the best way
of searching for these viruses.

At present, interpretation of the results obtained by direct EM of

faeces is not easy. The pathogenicity of most of the viruses described
here has not yet been adequately defined in the different animal species.
Furthermore, there is the probability that different strains of the same
virus may vary considerably in virulence. Although mixed infections occur
very frequently in the field, there has been very little experimental work
done using different combinations of viruses and mixed infections of
viruses and enteropathogenic bacteria. Detection of a virus in the faeces
of an animal with diarrhoea is therefore not sufficient grounds for
ascribing etiological significance to it. Results should be considered in
the light of bacteriological, and where possible, pathological findings.

When new virus-like particles are detected in faeces, the nature and
significance of such particles can only be assessed by answering the
following questions. How frequently are the particles detected in faeces?
Are they observed in material from normal animals as well as those with
diarrhoea? Does the period of their excretion coincide with that of
clinical symptoms? Is it possible to demonstrate an antibody response in
animals which have excreted the particles? Can they be isolated in cell
cultures, intestinal organ cultures etc? Are they capable of infecting
experimental animals, and if so, do such infections cause clinical disease?

REFERENCES

Appel, M.J.G., Cooper, B.J., Griesen, H. and Carmichael, L.E., 1978.
    Status report: canine viral enteritis. JAVMA, 173: 1516-1518.
Bass, E.P. and Sharpee, R.L., 1975. Coronavirus and gastroenteritis in
    foals. Lancet, ii: 822.
Bohl, E.H., 1979. Diagnosis of diarrhoea in pigs due to transmissable
    gastroenteritis virus or rotavirus. In: F. Bricout and R. Scherrer
    (Editors), Viral Enteritis in Humans and Animals. INSERM, Paris,
    pp. 341-343.
Caul, E.O., Paver, W.K. and Clarke, S.K.R., 1975. Coronavirus particles in
    faeces from patients with gastroenteritis. Lancet, i: 1192.
Caul, E.O. and Egglestone, S.I., 1979. Coronavirus-like particles present
    in simian faeces. Vet. Rec., 104: 168-169.
Chasey, D. and Cartwright, S.F., 1978. Virus-like particles associated
    with porcine epidemic diarrhoea. Res. Vet. Sci., 25: 255-256.
Eugster, A.K. and Nairn, C., 1977. Diarrhoea in puppies: parvovirus-like
    particles demonstrated in their faeces. Southwest Vet., 30: 59-60.
Eugster, A.K. and Sidwa, T., 1979. Rotaviruses in diarrhoeic faeces of a
    dog. Vet. Med. Sm. An. Clin., 74: 817-819.
Flewett, T.H., Bryden, A.S. and Davies, H., 1973. Virus particles in
    gastroenteritis. Lancet, ii: 1497.
Flewett, T.H., Bryden, A.S. and Davies, H., 1975. Virus diarrhoea in foals
    and other animals. Vet. Rec., 96: 477.
Flewett, T.H., Bryden, A.S., Davies, H. and Morris, C.A., 1975. Epidemic
    virus enteritis in a long-stay children's ward. Lancet, i: 4-5.

Flewett, T.H., 1978. Electron microscopy in the diagnosis of infectious
   diarrhoea. JAVMA, 173: 538-543.
Holmes, I.H., 1979. Viral gastroenteritis. In: J.L. Melnick (Editor),
   Progress in Medical Virology, 25: 1-36. Karger, Basel.
Hoshino, Y. and Scott, F.W., 1980. Coronavirus-like particles in the
   faeces of normal cats. Arch. Virol., 63: 147-152.
Kapikian, A.Z., Wyatt, R.G., Dolin, R., Thornhill, T.S., Kalica, A.R. and
   Chanock, R.M., 1972. Visualization by immune electron microscopy of a
   27 nm particle associated with acute infectious non-bacterial gastro-
   enteritis. J. Virol., 10: 1075-1081.
Madeley, C.R. and Cosgrove, B.P., 1975. Viruses in infantile gastroenteritis. Lancet, ii: 124.
Madeley, C.R. and Cosgrove, B.P., 1976. Caliciviruses in man. Lancet,
   i: 199-200.
Madeley, C.R., 1979. Comparison of the features of astroviruses and
   caliciviruses seen in samples of faeces by electron microscopy. J.
   infect. Dis., 139: 519-523.
Mathan, M., Mathan, V.I., Swaminathan, S.P., Yesudoss, S. and Baker, S.J.,
   1975. Pleomorphic virus-like particles in human faeces. Lancet, i:
   1068-1069.
McNulty, M.S., McFerran, J.B., Bryson, D.G., Logan, E.F. and Curran, W.L.,
   1976. Studies on rotavirus infection and diarrhoea in young calves.
   Vet. Rec., 99: 229-230.
McNulty, M.S., Curran, W.L., Todd, D. and McFerran, J.B., 1979a. Detection
   of viruses in avian faeces by direct electron microscopy. Avian
   Pathol., 8: 239-247.
McNulty, M.S., Allan, G.M., Todd, D. and McFerran, J.B., 1979b. Isolation
   and cell culture propagation of rotaviruses from turkeys and chickens.
   Arch. Virol., 61: 13-21.
McNulty, M.S., Curran, W.L. and McFerran, J.B., 1980. Detection of astro-
   viruses in turkey faeces by direct electron microscopy. Vet. Rec.,
   in press.
Mebus, C.A., Underdahl, N.R., Rhodes, M.B. and Twiehaus, M.J., 1969. Calf
   diarrhoea (scours): reproduced with a virus from a field outbreak.
   Univ. Neb. agric. exp. Station Res. Bull. No. 233.
Mebus, C.A., Rhodes, M.B. and Underdahl, N.R., 1978. Neonatal calf
   diarrhoea caused by a virus that induces villous epithelial cell
   syncitia. Am. J. Vet. Res., 39: 1223-1228.
Middleton, P.J., Szymanski, M.T. and Petric, M., 1977. Viruses associated
   with acute gastroenteritis in young children. Am. J. Dis. Child.,
   131: 733-737.
Pensaert, M.B. and de Bouck, P., 1978. A new coronavirus-like particle
   associated with diarrhoea in swine. Arch. Virol., 58: 243-247.
Ritchie, A.E., Desmukh, D.R., Larsen, C.T. and Pomeroy, B.S., 1973.
   Electron microscopy of coronavirus-like particles characteristic of
   turkey bluecomb disease. Avian Dis., 17: 546-558.
Rodger, S.M., Craven, J.A. and Williams, I., 1975. Demonstration of
   reovirus-like particles in intestinal contents of piglets with
   diarrhoea. Aust. Vet. J., 51: 536.
Saif, L.J., Bohl, E.H., Kohler, G.M. and Hughes, J.H., 1977. Immune
   electron microscopy of transmissable gastroenteritis virus and
   rotavirus (reovirus-like agent of swine). Am. J. Vet. Res., 38: 13-20.
Schnagl, R.D. and Holmes, I.H., 1978. Coronavirus-like particles in stools
   from dogs, from some country areas of Australia. Vet. Rec., 102:
   528-529.

10

Snodgrass, D.R., Smith, W., Gray, E.W. and Herring, J.A., 1976. A rotavirus
in lambs with diarrhoea. Res. Vet. Sci., 20: 113.
Snodgrass, D.R. and Gray, E.W., 1977. Detection and transmission of 30 nm
virus particles (astroviruses) in faeces of lambs with diarrhoea.
Arch. Virol., 55: 287-291.
Snodgrass, D.R., Angus, K.W. and Gray, E.W., 1979. A rotavirus from
kittens. Vet. Rec., 104: 222-223.
Stair, E.L., Rhodes, M.B., White, R.G. and Mebus, C.A., 1972. Neonatal calf
diarrhoea: purification and electron microscopy of a coronavirus-like
agent. Am. J. Vet. Res., 33: 1147-1156.
Storz, J. and Leary, J.J., 1979. Bovine parvoviruses: epidemiology and
host-virus relationships. In: F. Bricout and R. Scherrer (Editors),
Viral Enteritis in Humans and Animals. INSERM, Paris, pp. 63-80.
Tzipori, S., Smith, M. and Makin, T., 1978. Enteric coronavirus-like
particles in sheep. Aust. Vet. J., 54: 320-321.
Woode, G.N., Bridger, J.C., Jones, J.M., Flewett, T.H., Bryden, A.S.,
Davies, H.A. and White, G.B.B., 1976. Morphological and antigenic
relationships between viruses (rotaviruses) from acute gastroenteritis
of children, calves, piglets, mice and foals. Infect. Immun., 14:
804-810.
Woode, G.N. and Bridger, J.C., 1978. Isolation of small viruses resembling
astroviruses and caliciviruses from acute enteritis of calves. J.
Med. Microbiol., 11: 441-452.

Figs. 1-7. Viruses and virus-like particles detected in faeces by direct
electron microscopy. Bar represents 100 nm. Methylamine tungstate stain.
1. Bovine rotavirus. 2. Bovine enteric coronavirus. 3. Coronavirus-like
particles from simian faeces. 4. Turkey astrovirus. 5. Human calicivirus.
6. Canine parvovirus. 7. Porcine enterovirus-like particles.

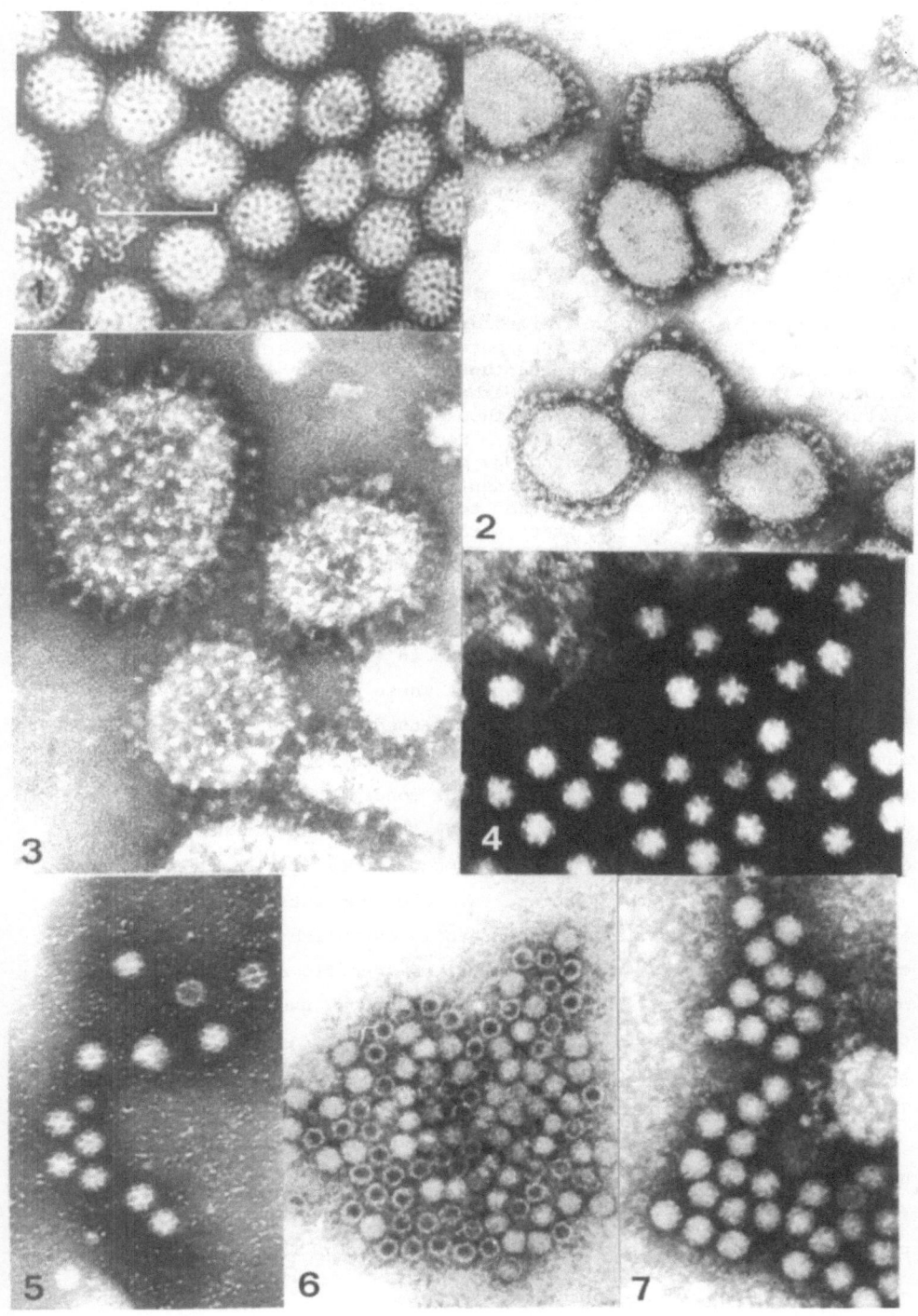

CELL CULTURE TECHNIQUES FOR THE IDENTIFICATION OF
ENTERIC VIRUSES - PRESENT POSSIBILITIES

J.C. Bridger

A.R.C. Institute for Research on Animal Diseases,
Compton, Nr. Newbury, Berkshire, U.K.

ABSTRACT

The current techniques available for the detection of transmissible
gastroenteritis virus, bovine and porcine rotaviruses, bovine enteric
coronavirus, bovine astrovirus and bovine parvovirus are reviewed.
Although, initially, the enteric pathogens were difficult to establish in
culture regularly, cell culture methods are currently available for
identification of several of them.   Some of the viruses can be detected
by serial passage with cytopathology but many techniques rely on the
production of antigens which are identified by immunofluorescent staining.
The techniques which have been used to detect serological differences
between the viruses and to detect viral antibody are reviewed and some of
the advantages and disadvantages of cell culture systems are discussed.

Cell culture techniques have played an insignificant role in the
discovery of viral enteric pathogens.   These agents do not appear to
replicate with cytopathology in commonly-used culture systems and without
doubt, this is one of the reasons why they were not identified earlier.
But, with increased understanding of the conditions necessary to infect
and demonstrate them in culture, cell culture techniques have become
available for the identification of some of these fastidious agents.

Although some of the viruses, the wild-type rotaviruses and
astroviruses in particular, do not readily establish a fully productive
cycle in cell cultures, they produce virus-specific antigens demonstrable
by immunofluorescence.   This property has proved useful for their
detection, even though serial passage could not be accomplished readily.

IDENTIFICATION OF ENTERIC VIRUSES

Transmissible gastroenteritis virus (TGEV)

This, the longest known viral enteric pathogen of calves or pigs,
has a history of being difficult to cultivate in cell cultures.   At
first, the virus was propagated in pig kidney cell cultures without the
production of a cytopathic effect (CPE) but during the period from 1963

to 1965 several workers were able to produce cytopathic effects in these cells with other strains, although production of a distinct CPE could require several passages (Reviewed by Bohl, 1975). Subsequently, inoculation of cell cultures from porcine thyroid or salivary glands produced more extensive cytopathic effects at the first passage and gave good results for isolation of TGEV. It has been suggested that, although they replicate in cell cultures, some strains do not readily produce a CPE even after several serial passages and Bohl (1979) described a cell culture-immunofluorescence test in swine testicular cells to detect such viruses. This test is similar to that used for rotaviruses and results can be obtained within 24 hours of inoculation. A plaque technique has also been described to detect and titrate TGEV.

Bohl (1975) commented that the choice of specimen for cell culture inoculation is important and that it should be derived from the jejunum of a young piglet, sick for less than 24 hours, as this can be expected to contain the highest concentration of virus. Some virus strains may not be readily isolated in cell cultures (M.B. Pensaert, personal communication to Woode, 1979) and thus where suitable material is available, immunofluorescent staining on gut sections may prove a more reliable technique.

Rotaviruses

In common with TGEV, the rotaviruses have a history of being difficult to cultivate by serial passage in cell cultures with cytopathology. However, Mebus et al. (1971) found that, although serial passage could not be accomplished readily, viral antigens could be detected by immunofluorescence in the cytoplasm of infected cells. Single fluorescing cells were seen but on serial passage these cells were usually lost. This cell culture-immunofluorescent test was used by Woode et al. (1974) and Meyling (1974) to detect the presence of bovine rotaviruses in experimental and field material. It provides a rapid result as the test can be read after incubation for 24 hours and results compared favourably to those obtained by electron microscopy (Bridger & Woode, 1975).

A similar cell culture-immunofluorescence test has been used for detection of porcine rotaviruses in both experimental and field material (McNulty et al., 1976; Woode et al., 1976; Bohl et al., 1978; Bohl, 1979). However, although the author has used this test to measure the

levels of six porcine rotaviruses in the faeces of experimental animals,
several investigators have reported that the number of infected cells
seen in cell cultures inoculated with field material is low even when
virus can be demonstrated by electron microscopy. Bohl (1979) has said
that his preferred method to detect porcine rotavirus is immunofluorescent
staining of mucosal scrapings.

Certain modifications to the cell culture-immunofluorescence test
can improve rotavirus isolation. Banatvala et al. (1975) first
described the use of centrifugation of infected monolayers to detect
human rotavirus and subsequently Chasey and Lucas (1977) showed that this
improved the number of cells infected with porcine rotavirus. With one
isolate of porcine rotavirus the author has shown that centrifugation of
infected monolayers at 300 g increases the level of infectious virus
0.5-1.0 $\log_{10}$ units. Two further modifications, one used by Ellens
et al. (1978) and the other by Babiuk et al. (1977) have improved
detection of bovine rotavirus. Compared to stationary cultures, Ellens
et al. scored more samples positive when cultures were rolled and the
number of cells showing fluorescence was greatly enhanced. Babiuk
et al. improved their ability to detect bovine rotaviruses by pretreating
faecal samples with trypsin. Thus, for maximum sensitivity, it would
appear that these modifications should be incorporated.

Only a small number of bovine rotaviruses had been passaged serially
in cell cultures until it was found that treatment with pancreatic
enzymes enhanced their cultivation. Serial passage of bovine
rotaviruses, sometimes with cytopathology, was shown to be more readily
accomplished when trypsin was added to the maintenance medium (Babiuk
et al., 1977; Almeida et al., 1978; Babiuk and Mohammed, 1978) and
Theil et al. (1977) reported similar findings for two porcine rotaviruses
using pancreatin. In these conditions rotaviruses can produce plaques
and a plaque technique for the isolation of bovine and porcine
rotaviruses from field material has been described (Bohl, 1979). Since
use has been made of enzymes in rotavirus cultivation, the number of
rotaviruses which can be serially passaged in cell cultures has increased
many times but it is not known whether all bovine and porcine rotaviruses
can be propagated by this technique and the sensitivity of rotavirus
detection by serial passage with trypsin remains to be evaluated.

Although much reliance has been placed on immunofluorescence to
detect rotaviruses in cell culture, it appears that some bovine

rotaviruses can be passaged serially with cytopathology without the addition of pancreatic enzymes. Isolations with obvious CPE in Northern Ireland (McNulty et al., 1977), Japan (Sato et al., 1978), and South Africa (Theodoridis et al., 1979) have been made and in some instances the cytopathic effect has been used to titrate the virus. Frey et al. (1979) claim to have isolated several cytopathogenic rotaviruses from faecal samples tested by serial passage in MDBK cells but electron microscopy detected more positive samples and no comparison was made with immunofluorescent staining of infected cultures.

Rotaviruses are not fastidious about the type of cell which they will infect; both primary cells and cell lines can be infected. For example, with the Cody isolate of bovine rotavirus, Fernelius et al. (1972) infected primary calf and lamb kidney, bovine embryonic trachea, bovine embryonic skin, Vero, mouse-L and PK-15 cell lines. Various monkey kidney cell lines have been popular: Thouless et al. (1977) infected LLC-MK$_2$ cells with rotaviruses from seven animal species, Bohl (1979) used MA-104 cells in a plaque technique and Babiuk et al. (1977) used BSC-1 cells for bovine rotavirus isolation in the presence of trypsin. MDBK (McNulty et al., 1977) and HeLa cells (Mebus et al., 1971) have also been infected with bovine rotaviruses.

Bovine enteric coronavirus

In contrast to the rotaviruses, a rapid cell culture-immunofluorescence test has not been used for demonstration of bovine coronavirus. Stott et al. (1976) first showed that an American cell-culture adapted strain would replicate in bovine tracheal organ cultures to produce haemagglutinating activity and immunofluorescent antigens. Subsequently, Bridger et al. (1978) applied this technique successfully to 'wild-type' coronaviruses present in faeces of experimental and field cases of the disease and the technique has been used successfully in other laboratories (Haralambiev et al., 1979; McNulty, personal communication). The results obtained agreed well with those obtained by electron microscopy and immunofluorescent staining of gut sections. The technique has also been used to isolate coronaviruses, identified by electron microscopy, from the bovine respiratory tract (Thomas et al., to be published).

Until recently, isolations in cell cultures were infrequent (Mebus et al., 1973; Bridger et al., 1978; Laporte et al., 1979) but two

recent reports offer hope of a cell culture diagnostic method.   A cell
line established from a human rectal adenocarcinoma (HRT-18 cells) has
been used for isolation of several bovine coronaviruses and produced
virus for up to at least 12 passages with titres in excess of 10^7 TCD_{50}
per ml (Laporte, 1980).   Secondly, Dea et al. (1980) isolated the virus
from intestinal contents in Vero cells with CPE.   They reported that
the pH of the inoculation and incubation medium influenced virus production, a factor shown to be important for isolation of other coronaviruses.

Bovine parvovirus

This virus has been associated with bovine enteritis by only one
group of workers (Storz and Bates, 1973).   Actively dividing cells are
required for its isolation and three methods have been described
(reviewed by Storz and Leary, 1979).   Cells may be cultured directly
from infected organs or serial passages can be made in actively growing
bovine foetal spleen cells.   Alternatively, inoculated spleen cells may
be passaged serially.   Parvovirus replication is demonstrated by the
production of haemagglutinating activity, cytopathic effects and nuclear
immunofluorescence and results obtained by cell culture isolation
correlated well with those from immunofluorescent staining of infected
tissues.

Bovine astroviruses

Although two isolates of bovine astrovirus failed to induce
diarrhoea in experimental calves (Woode and Bridger, 1978; Bridger and
Ormerod, unpublished observation), these viruses are of importance as
they may lead to an incorrect result from cell culture.   Antibody to
bovine astroviruses is common in bovine sera in the U.K. (Woode and
Bridger, 1978) and at this Institute over 90% of faeces collected from
calves up to 5 weeks of age contain astroviruses at up to 10^5 TCD_{50} per g
of faeces (E. Ormerod, personal communication).   Thus antisera produced
by inoculation of calves with faecal filtrates may contain antibody to
astroviruses in addition to antibody against an enteric pathogen.
Furthermore, when inoculated into bovine kidney cells and stained by
immunofluorescence, bovine astroviruses produce a similar pattern to the
rotaviruses; a point of difference is that fluorescent inclusions may
be seen in the nucleus.   Hence for correct identification by
immunofluorescence, freedom of antisera from astrovirus antibody must
be ensured.   This may be achieved by producing antisera to viruses

grown in cell cultures, as bovine astroviruses have not been propagated by serial passage in culture, but ideally the validity of the results should be assessed by confirmation with a serologically-independent test such as electron microscopy.

Other viruses

Some viruses for which there is evidence of a pathogenic role in neonatal diarrhoea still remain to be cultured in either cell or organ cultures.   These include the bovine calicivirus-like (Newbury) agents (Woode and Bridger, 1978;   Bridger and Hall, 1979), a bovine virus causing villus epithelial cell syncytia (Mebus et al., 1978) and a porcine coronavirus, CV777 (Pensaert and Debouck, 1978).

Identification of virus serotypes

When isolation can be made regularly in cell cultures, differences or similarities between virus isolates can be investigated.   Thus tests relying on the neutralization of cytopathic effects in cell cultures have shown that all isolates of TGEV are similar serologically (reviewed by Woode, 1969) and, apart from one Japanese strain, all isolates of bovine parvovirus appear identical to bovine parvovirus type 1 (Storz and Leary, 1979).

With viruses which cannot be serially propagated in vitro, serological differences may still be established by cell culture techniques.   For example, Thouless et al. (1977) differentiated rotaviruses from several animal species using a fluorescent focus reduction test.   This test relies on the ability of rotaviruses to infect cells without releasing infectious virus and, in the author's laboratory, has differentiated between rotaviruses from the bovine population.   With rotaviruses adapted to serial passage and plaque production, Estes and Graham (1980) used a plaque reduction test to distinguish between simian, porcine and bovine rotaviruses.

There have been no reports concerning the serological homogeneity or otherwise of the bovine enteric coronaviruses but, presumably, this could be investigated with viruses isolated in tracheal organ cultures, HRT-18 or Vero cells.

DETECTION OF ANTIBODY TO ENTERIC VIRUSES

Where cell culture systems exist, specific antibody may be demonstrated by neutralization of virus effects or by staining infected cultures by an indirect immunofluorescent antibody test.

Neutralization tests, relying on inhibition of cytopathic effects or plaque reduction, are useful for the detection of TGEV antibodies (reviewed by Bohl, 1975).

Immunofluorescent staining of cell cultures by the indirect technique is made possible when cell-culture adapted strains become available and the existence of only a few adapted strains has been useful. The indirect immunofluorescence technique can also be applied to viruses which show limited multiplication in cell cultures, for example the rotaviruses and astroviruses. The usefulness of serological detection of the endemic enteric viruses - the rotaviruses and corona- viruses - is limited, however, because of the high levels of passively- acquired antibody in farm animals.

GENERAL REMARKS AND CONCLUSIONS

In a sphere where viruses are commonly identified by electron microscopy, multiplication of an agent in cell cultures confirms that the agent is one capable of replication in mammalian cells. This is particularly useful for enveloped viruses, such as coronaviruses, which may be confused with cellular debris in the electron microscope but also rules out the possibility that the particles observed might be bacteriophages.

Multiplication of a virus in cell cultures enables stocks of viruses to be prepared so that viruses isolated at different times and locations can be compared. It also offers a means of purifying viruses by plaque or terminal dilution methods and a means of quantifying viruses.

As only infectious virus will be measured, viral sub-units or virus which has lost infectivity will not, in contrast to other tests such as complement fixation or ELISA tests. Cell culture techniques are at a disadvantage if all strains of a virus are not cultured readily, as has been suggested for TGEV, and these viruses will be missed unless alternative techniques are used. Although cell culture-adapted viruses have been useful, when only a minority of viruses can be cultured, there is a danger that those isolated might not be typical.

As a group, the enteric viruses have not been cultured readily but we may conclude that by providing correct conditions, methods for detection and isolation of several of them have become available. Many of the techniques rely on immunofluorescent staining and the mono- specificity of the working antisera is then essential. This can

be checked by a technique such as electron microscopy which does not rely
on serology.

REFERENCES

Almeida, J.D., Hall, T., Banatvala, J.E., Totterdell, B.M. and
Chrystie, I.L.: The effect of trypsin on the growth of rotavirus.
J. gen. Virol. 40: 213-218, 1978.
Babiuk, L.A. and Mohammed, K.A.: Trypsin and bovine rotavirus
replication. Vet. Rec. 102: 61-62, 1978.
Babiuk, L.A., Mohammed, K., Spence, L., Fauvel, M. and Petro, R.:
Rotavirus isolation and cultivation in the presence of trypsin.
J. clin. Microbiol. 6: 610-617, 1977.
Banatvala, J.E., Totterdell, B., Chrystie, I.L. and Woode, G.N.:
In vitro detection of human rotaviruses. Lancet, ii: 821, 1975.
Bohl, E.H.: Transmissible gastroenteritis. Diseases of Swine, Fourth
Edition, Ed. H.W. Dunne and A.D. Leman. pp 168-188 (Iowa State
University Press, Ames, Iowa, USA, 1975).
Bohl, E.H.: Diagnosis of diarrhea in pigs due to transmissible
gastroenteritis virus or rotavirus. INSERM 90: 341-344, 1979.
Bohl, E.H., Kohler, E.M., Saif, L.J., Cross, R.F., Agnes, A.G. and
Theil, K.W.: Rotavirus as a cause of diarrhea in pigs. J. Amer.
vet. med. Assoc. 172: 458-463, 1978.
Bridger, J.C. and Hall, G.A.: Effects of a calicivirus-like agent (the
Newbury agent) on gnotobiotic calves. INSERM 90: 233-236, 1979.
Bridger, J.C. and Woode, G.N.: Neonatal calf diarrhoea: Identification
of a reovirus-like (rotavirus) agent in faeces by immunofluorescence
and immune electron microscopy. Br. vet. J. 131: 528-535, 1975.
Bridger, J.C., Woode, G.N., Meyling, A.: Isolation of coronaviruses from
neonatal calf diarrhoea in Great Britain and Denmark. Vet.
Microbiol. 3: 101-113, 1978.
Chasey, D. and Lucas, M. Detection of rotavirus in experimentally
infected piglets. Res. vet. Sci. 22: 124-125, 1977.
Dea, S., Roy, R.S., Begin, M.E.: Bovine coronavirus isolation and
cultivation in continuous cell lines. Amer. J. vet. Res. 41:
30-38, 1980.
Ellens, D.J., de Leeuw, P.W., Straver, P.J. and van Balkan, J.A.M.:
Comparison of five diagnostic methods for the detection of rotavirus
antigens in calf faeces. Med. Microbiol. Immunol. 166: 157-163,
1978.
Estes, M.K. and Graham, D.Y.: Identification of rotaviruses of different
origins by the plaque-reduction test. Amer. J. vet. Res. 41:
151-152, 1980.
Fernelius, A.L., Ritchie, A.E., Classick, L.G., Norman, J.O. and
Mebus, C.A.: Cell culture adaptation and propagation of a reovirus-
like agent of calf diarrhea from a field outbreak in Nebraska.
Arch. ges. Virusforsch. 37: 114-130, 1972.
Frey, H.R., Marschall, H.J. and Liess, B.: Rotavirusinfektionen in
norddeutschen Kälberbeständen : Nachweis mittels Elektronen-
mikroskopie und Virusanzüchtung in Zellkuren. Dtsch. tierärztl.
Wschr 86: 100-104, 1979.
Haralambiev, H.E., Mitov, B.K. and Popov, G.V.: Isolation of bovine
corona and rotaviruses in organ cultures from respiratory mucosa.
Comptes rendus de l'Academie bulgare des Sciences 32: 1597-1600,
1979.

20

Laporte, J., Bobulesco, P. and Rossi, F.: Une lignée cellulaire
    particulièrement sensible à la replication du Coronavirus
    entéritique bovin : les cellules HRT 18.   C.R. Acad. Sc, t. 290:
    Série D 623-626, 1980.
Laporte, J., L'Haridon, R. and Bobulesco, P.: In vitro culture of bovine
    enteritic coronavirus (BEC).   INSERM 90: 99-102, 1979.
McNulty, M.S., Allan, G.M. and McFerran, J.B.: Cell culture studies with
    a cytopathic bovine rotavirus.   Arch. Virol. 54: 201-209, 1977.
McNulty, M.S., Pearson, G.R., McFerran, J.B., Collins, D.S. and
    Allan, G.M.: A reovirus-like agent (rotavirus) associated with
    diarrhoea in neonatal pigs.   Vet. Microbiol. 1: 55-63, 1976.
Mebus, C.A., Kono, M., Underdahl, N.R. and Twiehaus, M.J.: Cell culture
    propagation of neonatal calf diarrhea (scours) virus.   Can. vet. J.
    12: 69-72, 1971.
Mebus, C.A., Rhodes, M.B., Underdahl, M.S.: Neonatal calf diarrhea
    caused by a virus that induces villous epithelial cell syncytia.
    Amer. J. vet. Res. 39: 1223-1228, 1978.
Mebus, C.A., Stair, E.L., Rhodes, M.B. and Twiehaus, M.S.: Neonatal
    calf diarrhea : propagation, attenuation and characteristics of a
    coronavirus-like agent.   Amer. J. vet. Res. 34: 145-150, 1973.
Meyling, A.: Reo-like neonatal calf diarrhoea (NCD) virus demonstrated
    in Denmark.   Acta vet. scand. 15: 457-459, 1974.
Pensaert, M.B. and Debouck, P.: A new coronavirus-like particle
    associated with diarrhea in swine.   Arch. Virol. 58: 243-247, 1978.
Sato, K., Inaba, Y., Takahashi, E., Ito, Y., Kurogi, H., Akashi, H.,
    Satoda, K., Omori, T. and Matumoto, M.: Isolation of a reovirus-like
    agent (rotavirus) from neonatal calf diarrhea in Japan.   Microbiol.
    Immunol. 22: 499-503, 1978.
Storz, J. and Bates, R.C.: Parvovirus infections in calves.   J. Amer.
    vet. med. Assoc. 163: 884-886, 1973.
Storz, J. and Leary, J.J.: Bovine parvoviruses : epidemiology and
    host-virus relationships.   INSERM 90: 63-80, 1979.
Stott, E.J., Thomas, L.H., Bridger, J.C. and Jebbett, N.J.: Replication
    of a bovine coronavirus in organ cultures of foetal trachea.
    Vet. microbiol. 1: 65-69, 1976.
Theil, K.W., Bohl, E.H. and Agnes, A.G.: Cell culture propagation of
    porcine rotavirus (reovirus-like agent).   Amer. J. vet. Res. 38:
    1765-1768, 1977.
Theodoridis, A., Prozesky, L. and Els, H.J.: The isolation and
    cultivation of calf rotavirus in the Republic of South Africa.
    Onderstepoort J. vet. Res. 46: 65-69, 1979.
Thouless, M.E., Bryden, A.S., Flewett, T.H., Woode, G.N., Bridger, J.C.,
    Snodgrass, D.R. and Herring, J.A.: Serological relationships
    between rotaviruses from different species as studied by complement
    fixation and neutralization.   Arch. Virol. 53: 287-294, 1977.
Woode, G.N.: Transmissible gastroenteritis of swine.   Vet. Bull. 39:
    239-248, 1969.
Woode, G.N.: Viral infections of the intestinal tract : pathological
    and clinical aspects.   INSERM 90: 15-38, 1979.
Woode, G.N. and Bridger, J.C.: Isolation of small viruses resembling
    astroviruses and caliciviruses from acute enteritis of calves.
    J. med. Microbiol. 11: 441-452, 1978.
Woode, G.N., Bridger, J.C., Hall, G. and Dennis, M.J.: The isolation of
    a reovirus-like agent associated with diarrhoea in colostrum-
    deprived calves in Great Britain.   Res. vet. Sci. 16: 102-105,
    1974.

Woode, G.N., Bridger, J.C., Hall, G.A., Jones, J.M. and Jackson, G.:
    The isolation of reovirus-like agents (rotaviruses) from acute
    gastroenteritis of piglets.   J. med. Micro. 9:   203-209, 1976.

DIAGNOSIS BY ENZYME-LINKED IMMUNOSORBENT ASSAY

Daniel J. Ellens[1]

Central Veterinary Institute, Department of Virology,

39 Houtribweg, NL 8221 RA Lelystad, the Netherlands.

ABSTRACT

A variety of enzyme-linked immunosorbent assay (ELISA) systems are being applied in the detection and quantification of both antibodies and antigens in bacterial, viral and parasitic infections. To date, the use of ELISA in research on neonatal diarrhoea has been described for the detection of rotavirus, bovine coronavirus and enteropathogenic *Escherichia coli* infections.

Some features of the double antibody sandwich ELISA system are discussed with particular reference to those elements most important in determining the specificity and sensitivity of the test.

INTRODUCTION

About 10 years ago Van Weemen and Schuurs (1971) and Engvall and Perlmann (1971) introduced enzyme-labeled probes for immunological assay purposes. The novel approach appeared to have distinct advantages over conventional immunological tests. Its sensitivity was comparable to radioimmunoassay and yet it missed the drawbacks of the latter technique. In fact ELISA seemed to provide all the elements for an ideal immunoassay: safe, sensitive, easy to perform, inexpensive, utilizing a tracer molecule with great stability, not requiring sophisticated equipment and suited for automation.

Perhaps the major area in which enzyme-linked immunosorbent assays emerge as the best substitutes for other assay systems, is in large scale screening programmes for various antigens or antibodies, especially in those situations where only qualitative information is needed. Systems making use of microplates are particularly well suited for this purpose. In many cases, simple visual observation of the enzyme-mediated reaction is adequate. Some ELISA screening systems have been completely automated (Ruitenberg et al., 1977). In recent years ELISA has been successfully

[1] Present address: Organon Teknika B.V., Department Membranes & Adsorption Stationsplein 1, 5281 GH Boxtel, the Netherlands.

employed not only in sero-epidemiology for bacterial, viral or parasitic human diseases, but also for agricultural and veterinary mass surveys (Clark and Adams, 1977; De Leeuw et al., 1980).

TYPES OF ASSAY

Two basic systems have been developed for enzyme immunoassays: blocking systems and trapping systems.

Blocking systems. Fig. 1a shows the principle of a blocking test for the detection of antigen. The antigen to be detected competes with a known quantity of enzyme-labeled (standard) antigen for a limited amount of specific antibody. The difference in optical density between control wells, containing only labeled antigen, and wells containing both standard antigen and test samples, is used to estimate the quantity of antigen present. This design of ELISA has to be used when the antigen possesses only one antigenic site (hapten). A similar system can be applied for the detection of antibody (figs. 1b and 1c). The advantage of this method for the detection of antibody is that antibodies of different species, directed against the same antigen(s), can be detected and quantitated using the same assay. For instance, bovine, porcine, human and simian sera have been examined by one blocking assay for the presence of antibodies against group-specific rotavirus antigens (Yolken et al., 1978).

The ELISA-inhibition technique, as shown in Fig. 1d, may also be listed under this heading. The test measures the ability of putative antigen-containing specimens to inhibit the binding of a limited amount of antiviral antibody to bound viral antigen. This assay does not require the use of high titered antiviral antisera in contrast with all other enzyme immunoassays for the detection of antigens. It has been described for the detection of Candida antigen in sera (Segal et al., 1979) and influenza virus in nasal washings (Berg et al., 1980).

Trapping system. The most widely used method for the detection of antibody is the indirect enzyme immunoassay (Fig. 2a). The method requires purified antigen and a conjugate that should be free of antibodies against the antigen. In principle the method permits the use of a single anti-species conjugate for the detection of antibodies against different agents. In addition, class-specific antibody activity may be measured by using appropriate conjugates. However, competition between antibodies of different classes may lead to a blocking effect: small amounts of anti-rotavirus IgA, for instance, may not be detected in the presence of a large excess of anti-rotavirus IgG.

The double antibody sandwich method (Fig. 2b) has been applied for the detection of a variety of high molecular weight antigens such as viruses and bacterial components. The method requires high titered specific antibody for trapping the antigen. The trapped antigen can be detected either directly or indirectly (Figs. 2b and 2c). The latter method requires antigen-specific antibodies prepared in two different species. However, neither of these have to be conjugated.

The indirect double antibody sandwich method can also be used for the detection of class-specific antibody (Fig. 2d). First, the specific class of antibody is trapped and incubated with antigen. Bound antigen is then detected by the appropriate conjugate. The advantage of this design is that competition between different classes of antibody does not occur.

Instead of using specific antibody, the solid phase can also be coated with specific receptors (Figs. 2e and 2f). For instance, the ganglioside GM 1 has been used by Svennerholm and Holmgren (1978) to trap heat-labile enterotoxin.

THE DOUBLE ANTIBODY SANDWICH TECHNIQUE

The detection and quantification of antigen by the double antibody sandwich technique is usually done in four steps:
1. coating of the solid phase with antibody,
2. incubation of the coated surface with putative antigen containing samples,
3. incubation with specific antibody enzyme conjugate, and
4. estimation of bound conjugate activity.

Some points of importance to obtain optimal results with the double antibody sandwich ELISA are discussed below.

Preparation of specific antisera. Specificity and sensitivity of this type of assay are highly dependent on the availability of high titered antisera possessing high specificity. Usually such sera are prepared by hyperimmunization of rabbits, guinea pigs or goats with purified antigen. Prerequisites are that the animals have very low pre-immunization antibody levels, that the antigen preparation used for hyperimmunization is free of contaminating proteins and that the appropriate antigenic determinants are present. With rotavirus, for instance, purification procedures using CsCl centrifugation may damage the outer capside antigenic determinants (Kalica et al., 1977). Similar problems are well-known in the purification of coronaviruses. However, loss of coronavirus peplomers can be prevented by glutardialdehyde fixation during sucrose gradient rate zonal centrifugation of the virus (Dr. D. van Zaane, pers. comm.).

Due to the presence of immune complexes, antigens isolated from faeces are often contaminated with antibody. Use of these antigen preparations for hyperimmunization may lead to antiglobulin antibodies which interfere in the ELISA. This problem may be circumvented by hyperimmunizing orally infected newborn animals with antigen prepared from their own faeces (Ellens et al., 1978). Sera prepared by inoculation of rabbits with immune precipitates obtained by cross-immunoelectrophoresis of purified rotavirus against rabbit-anti-rotavirus serum are also suited for use in ELISA (Grauballe, these proceedings).

Coating of the solid phase. In general proteins adsorb to solid phases by either polar or apolar interactions. Polar interactions dominate the adsorption process at hydrophilic surfaces. Such interactions are sensitive to changes in environmental conditions so that proteins often can be removed from hydrophilic surfaces by exposure to extreme pH, high ionic strength or by extensive rinsing. At hydrophobic surfaces the adsorption process is dominated by apolar interactions. Hydrophobic regions of the protein surface are attached to the sorbent. The affinity between a given protein and a sorbent surface increases with increasing hydrophobicity of that surface. Desorption from hydrophobic surfaces usually does not occur. Protein adsorption isotherms generally develop well established plateau values that range between, say, 1 and 5 mg/m^2, corresponding to closely packed monolayers (Norde, 1980). For ELISA purposes, generally a tenfold lower adsorbed protein concentration is used. Too high a concentration of protein during coating may give rise to high background values or prozone phenomena. If the protein concentration used for coating is too low, the sensitivity of the ELISA will decrease. It is therefore essential to establish the optimal concentration for coating in each antibody-antigen system.

In view of the facts mentioned above, hydrophobic surfaces should be used as solid phase in ELISA, in spite of the given that hydrophilic surfaces absorb some proteins more efficiently at low concentrations.

Optimal adsorption at hydrophobic surfaces occurs around the isoelectric point of the protein, although for some proteins, e.g. - globulins, the optimal pH range is rather broad. Thus, when total serum is used for coating a solid phase with antibody, a pH of 9.5 is advantagous, because at this pH most contaminating serum proteins are adsorbed with low efficiency, whereas the coating efficiency of IgG is only slightly lower than at pH 7.2. However, to prevent non-specific reactions the use of purified reagents for coating is to be preferred. Neither the time nor the temperature of incubation appears to be very critical. Several hours at 4-37°C are used generally. When, during incubation, the tubes or plates are rotated at an angle, a larger surface area is coated. Coated plates or tubes have a long shelf life (more than one year) when stored between -20°C and +4°C.

Washing procedure. Several procedures can be used for washing plates or tubes between successive incubation steps. Generally the individual wells or tubes are washed with a 0.05% Tween solution by three cycles of filling and sucking-off. Reproducible results have also been obtained by rinsing microplates by immersing them in a washing solution (Grauballe, these proceedings) and by the use of a 96-channel shower device (Ellens, these proceedings).

Incubation with antigen. Depending on the antigen, incubation may be done at 4°C or at 37°C in order to reduce the reaction time. In the presence of excess antigen the antigen-antibody reaction in ELISA is virtually completed within half an hour. At more diluted antigen concentrations several hours of incubation may be needed to obtain an appropriate degree of antigen binding. It must, however, be kept in mind that detachment phenomena may occur.

To prepare test samples from faecal material, simple homogenization in several volumes of phosphate buffered saline usually suffices. Clarification or filtration of the homogenates may remove antigen aggregates.

Arklone extraction has been used to disrupt immune complexes in the faeces (Ellens et al., 1978). Reproducibility may be improved by adjusting the pH of the extract using phenol-red as an indicator (Middleton et al., 1977).

Conjugate. The enzymes Horse Radish Peroxidase (HRP) and Alkaline Phosphatase (AP) are most widely used in the preparation of ELISA conjugates. HRP is relatively cheap and is coupled quite efficiently to antibodies by the method of Wilson and Nakane (1978). Orthophenylenediamine (OPD) and 5-aminosalicylic acid (5-AS) are both suitable HRP substrates, although 5-AS has some advantages over OPD (Gielkens, these proceedings). Paranitro-phenylphosphate is generally used as AP substrate. There is no

significant difference between the sensitivity of ELISAs using AP or HRP. Recently, it has been reported that use of fluorescent or tritiated AP substrates increases the sensitivity of ELISA 100 to 1,000-fold. However, these substrates do not allow visual reading (Harris et al., 1979).
At high conjugate concentrations the binding is rapid and may be completed within half an hour. However, the use of high conjugate concentrations is expensive and may lead to high background values. Therefore the minimum concentration of a given conjugate needed for optimal results has to be determined by checkerboard titration. At the optimal conjugate concentration, incubation for 2-4 hours is usually sufficient.

Reading. Most systems in use for determining enzyme activity utilize a substrate that is converted to a coloured product which can be estimated photometrically (Gielkens, these proceedings). To determine the absolute concentration of antigen, a reference, in which the antigen content has been determined with another assay, is needed. For routine antigen determination a relative quantification of the antigen concentration in terms of ELISA units is often more convenient.

Design of confirmation reactions. In general there are two different systems to confirm the specificity of a double antibody sandwich test:
i. coating the solid phase with a pre-immune serum in parallel with hyperimmune serum (Fig. 3a) and ii. blocking the detection reaction (conjugate binding) by prior incubation with a known positive serum, preferably a convalescent serum of an experimentally infected gnotobiotic animal (Fig. 3b). By coating the solid phase with a pre-immune serum, the *physical specificity* of the reaction is investigated; i.e. non-specific adsorption can be excluded. The *immunological specificity* of the reaction is not confirmed since the hyperimmune serum may contain antibodies directed against other antigens (Fig. 3a). For this purpose the blocking test, as mentioned previously, has to be performed (Fig. 3b). The physical specificity of the reaction can also be confirmed by the use of pre-immune serum as blocking serum. Mentioned pre-immune serum can also be added directly to the conjugate as a carrier protein.

28

REFERENCES

Berg, R.A., Rennard, S.I., Murphy, B.R., Yolken, R.H., Dolin, R. and Straus, S.E.: New enzyme immunoassays for measurement of influenza A/Victoria/ 3/75/ virus in nasal washes. The Lancet, vol. I: 851-853, 1980.

Clark, M.F. and Adams, A.N.: Characteristics of the microplate method of enzyme-linked immunosorbent assay for the detection of plant viruses. J. Gen. Virol. 34: 475-483, 1977.

De Leeuw, P.W., Ellens, D.J., Straver, P.J., Van Balken, J.A.M., Moerman, A. and Baanvinger, Th.: Rotavirus infection in calves in dairy herds. Res.Vet.Sci. 29: 135-141, 1980.

Ellens, D.J., De Leeuw, P.W., Straver, P.J. and Van Balken, J.A.M.: Comparison of five diagnostic methods for the detection of rotavirus antigens in calf faeces. Med.Microbiol.Immunol. 166: 157-163, 1978.

Engvall, E. and Perlman, P.: Enzyme-linked immunosorbent assay (ELISA). Quantitative assay of immunoglobulin G. Immunochemistry 8: 871, 1971.

Harris, C.C., Yolken, R.H., Krokan, H. and Hsu, I.C.: Ultrasensitive enzymatic radioimmunoassay: Application to detection of cholera toxin and rotavirus. Proc. Natl. Acad. Sci. U.S.A. 76: 5336-5339, 1979.

Kalica, A.R., Purcell, R.H., Sereno, M.M., Wyatt, R.G., Kim, H.W., Channock, R.M. and Kapikian, A.J.: A microtiter solid phase radioimmunoassay for the detection of the human reovirus-like agent in stools. J.Immun. 118: 1275-1279, 1977.

Norde, W.: Adsorption of proteins at solid surfaces. In: Adhesion and adsorption of polymers. Polymer science and technology, vol. 12B, Plenum Press, N.Y., Lieng Huang Lee ed., p. 801, 1980.

Ruitenberg, E.J., Van Amstel, J.A., Brosi, B.J.M. and Steerenberg, P.A.: Mechanization of the enzyme-linked immunosorbent assay (ELISA) for large scale screening of sera. J.Immunol.Meth. 16: 351-359, 1977.

Segal, E., Berg, R.A., Pizzo, P. and Bennett, J.E.: Detection of candida antigen in sera of patients with candiasis by an enzyme-linked immunosorbent assay-inhibition technique. J.Clin.Microbiol. 10: 116-119, 1979.

Svennerholm, A.M. and Holmgren, J.: Identification of *E. coli* heat-labile enterotoxin (LT) by means of a ganglioside immunosorbent assay (Gm1-ELISA). Current Microbiology, 1: 19-24, 1978.

Van Weemen, B.K. and Schuurs, A.H.W.M.: Immunoassay using antigen-enzyme conjugates. FEBS Lett. 15: 232-236, 1971.

Wilson, B. and Nakane, P.K.: Recent developments in the periodate method of conjugating horseradish peroxidase (HRPO) to antibodies. In: Immunofluorescence and related staining techniques. Elsevier/North-Holland Biomedical Press. W. Knapp, K. Holubar and G. Wicks, eds., p. 215, 1978.

Yolken, R.H., Barbour, B., Wyatt, R.G., Kalica, A.R., Kapikian, A.Z. and Channock, R.M.: Enzyme-linked immunosorbent assay for identification of rotaviruses from different animal species. Science 201: 259-262, 1978.

LEGEND TO THE FIGURES
  1. Schematic representation of blocking methods for the detection of antibody or antigen.
a. competition between labelled and unlabelled antigen
b, c. competition between labelled and unlabelled antibody
d. inhibition method for the detection of antigen (antibody combining methods).
Asterisk denotes antigen or antibody to be detected.
  2. Schematic representation of trapping methods for the detection of antibody or antigen.
a. indirect method for detection of antibody
b. double antibody sandwich method for the detection of antigen
c, d. indirect double antibody sandwich method for the detection of antigen and antibody, respectively
e, f. alternative sandwich methods.
Asterisk denotes antigen or antibody to be detected.
  3. Schematic representation of confirmation methods.
a. coating with pre-immune serum (⊸)
b. blocking of the conjugate binding with a specific convalescent phase serum.
  ⊸ denotes contaminating antibody present in immune sera. Asterisk denotes antigen to be detected.

30

Fig 1

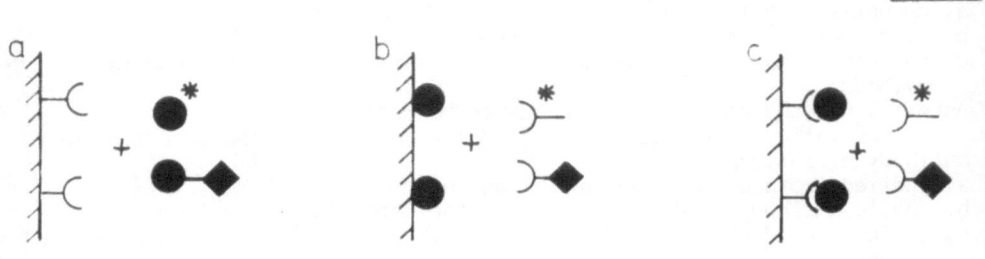

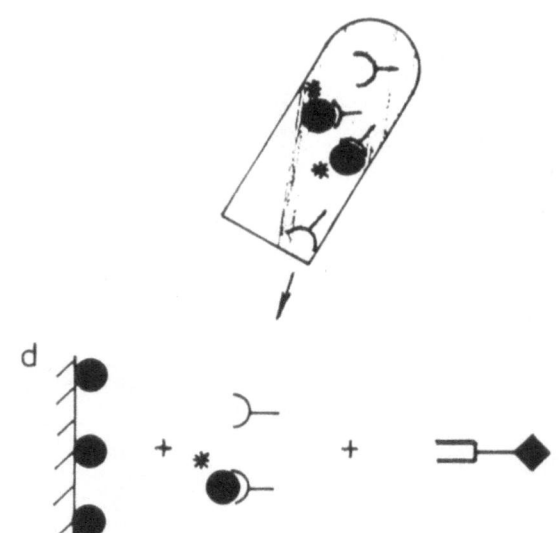

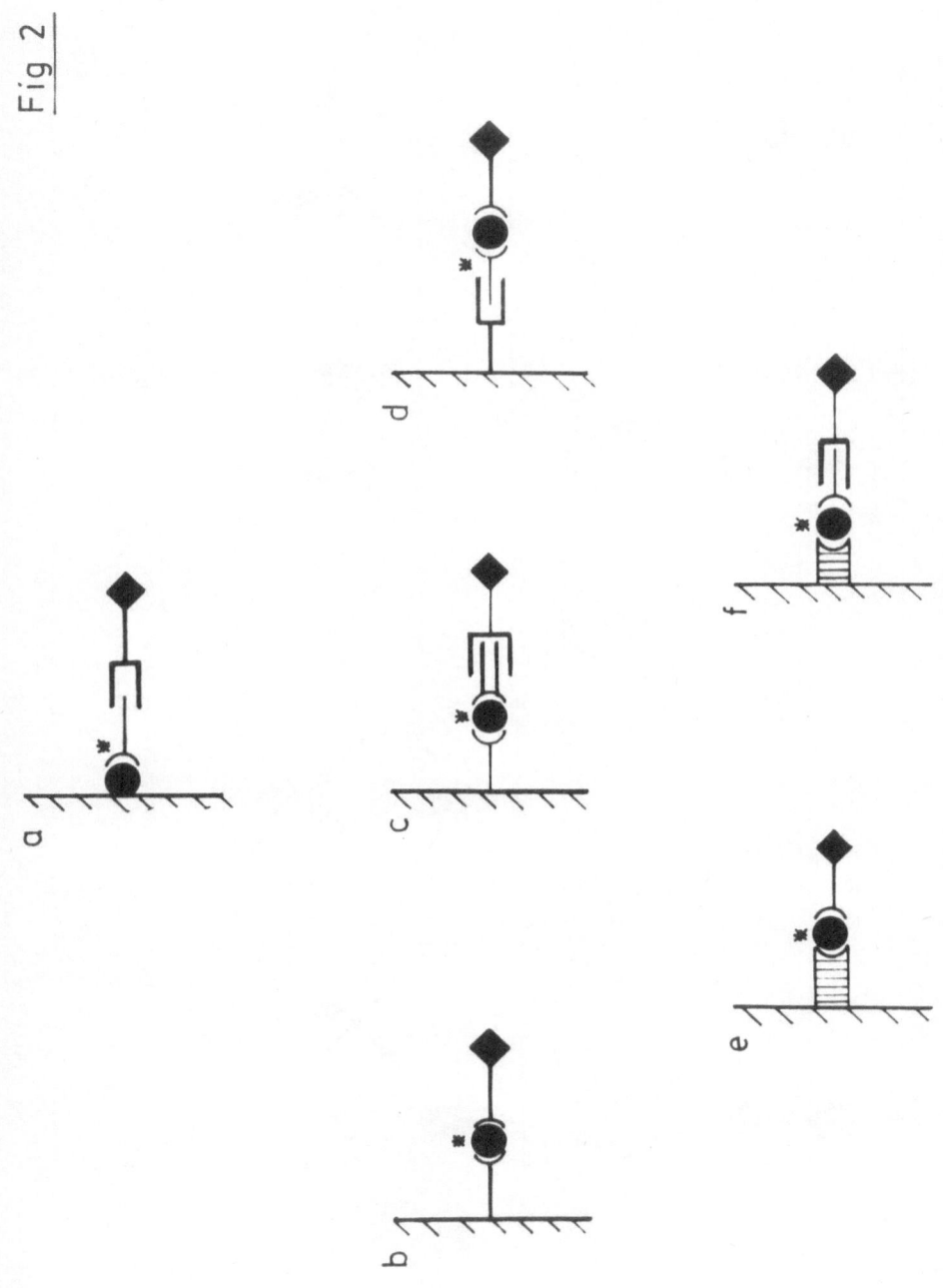

Fig 2

Fig 3

a

b

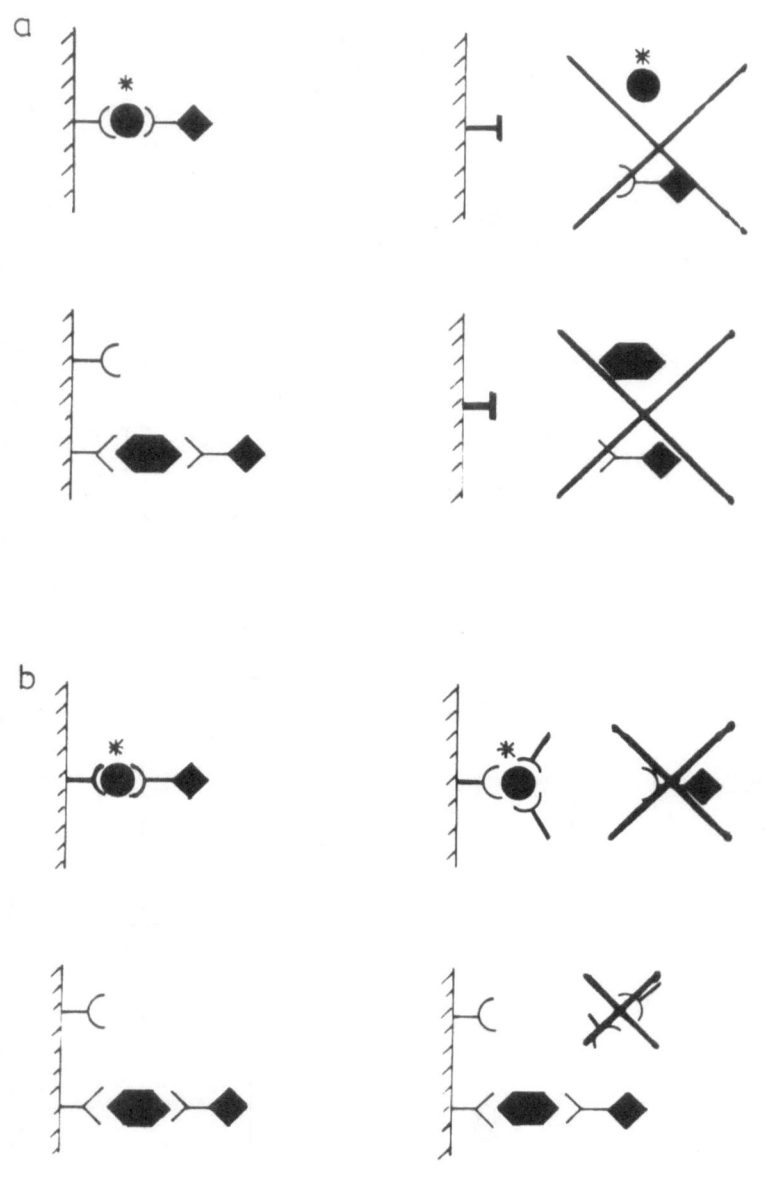

APPLICATION OF PURIFIED 5-AMINOSALICYLIC ACID AS SUBSTRATE IN ENZYME-LINKED IMMUNOSORBENT ASSAY (ELISA)

Arno L.J. Gielkens and Daniel J. Ellens[1]

Central Veterinary Institute, Department of Virology,

39, Houtribweg, NL 8221 RA Lelystad, the Netherlands.

ABSTRACT

Commercially available 5-aminosalicylic acid (5-AS) was recrystallised in the presence of $Na_2S_2O_5$. A completely colourless solution was obtained when the purified product was dissolved at a concentration of 1 mg/ml in a phosphate buffer containing EDTA and H_2O_2. No significant increase in absorption was found upon storage for 18 h at 4°C.

An 8-fold increase in sensitivity of an enzyme-linked immunosorbent assay for the detection of rotavirus antigens was demonstrated by using purified instead of commercially available 5-AS. In addition, P/N values did not significantly change between 2 and 18 h after addition of the substrate, thus rendering the time of reading less critical. No difference in sensitivity of the assay was found when comparing the modified 5-AS solution and ortho-phenylenediamine (OPD) as substrate. However, since OPD requires special care in handling, the modified 5-AS solution is preferred for use in routine ELISAs.

INTRODUCTION

Several substrates are available for use in enzyme immunoassays that employ horseradish peroxidase as the enzyme label. Ortho-phenylenediamine (OPD) has been reported as the most sensitive substrate for detecting minute quantities of the enzyme, but requires special care in handling because of its photosensitive and mutagenic properties (Ames et al., 1975; Voller et al., 1979). The widely used peroxidase substrate, 5-amino-salicylic acid (5-AS), does not pose these problems (Voogd et al., 1980). However, its solubility is limited and a solution of commercially available 5-AS in water is not colourless. Furthermore colour intensity increases with storage. For these reasons attempts were made to purify commercially available 5-AS for use in routine ELISAs.

[1]Present address: Organon Teknika B.V., Membranes and Adsorption Department, Stationsplein 1, NL 5281 GH Boxtel, the Netherlands.

MATERIALS AND METHODS

Purification of 5-aminosalicylic acid (5-AS)

Nine g of 5-AS (5-amino-2-hydroxybenzoic acid, Merck) and 9 g of sodium bisulphite ($Na_2S_2O_5$, Merck) were dissolved in 1 l demineralised water at $80°C$. To this solution, 4 g of charcoal were added; it was stirred for 5 min and then filtered. The filtrate was rapidly cooled to $4°C$ and the resulting white precipitate was collected by filtration through filter paper in a Buchner funnel. The residue was washed twice with 50 ml demineralised water at $4°C$, collected, dried and stored in the dark at room temperature.

Conventional 5-AS substrate solution

5-AS substrate solutions were prepared as described by Ruitenberg et al. (1975). Unless otherwise indicated, 10 mg of 5-AS were dissolved in 10 ml demineralised water of $70°C$; the pH of this solution was brought to 5.95 ($22°C$) with 1 N NaOH. Just before use, 1 ml 0.05% hydrogen peroxide was added to 9 ml of the freshly prepared 5-AS solution.

Modified 5-AS substrate solution

Stock 5-AS substrate solutions were prepared by dissolving 1 g of purified 5-AS in 1 l of substrate buffer composed of 2.6 vols. of 0.01 M NaH_2PO_4 (Merck), 2.75 vols. of 0.01 M Na_2HPO_4 (Merck) and 0.05 vols. of 0.01 M Na_2EDTA (Merck), pH 6.8. The final pH of this substrate solution varies between 5.9 and 6.0. Ten to 50 ml portions of this solution were stored at $-20°C$ until use. After thawing, the minute precipitate was dissolved at $37°C$ and subsequently 0.1 ml of 0.5% hydrogen peroxide was added per 10 ml of substrate solution. The pH of a substrate solution with a 5-AS concentration not equal to 1 mg/ml was adjusted to 5.95 before adding the hydrogen peroxide.

OPD substrate solution

The OPD substrate solution (ingredients kindly provided by Dr. W. Duermeyer, Organon, Oss, the Netherlands) was prepared according to Wolters et al. (1976). It consisted of phosphate-citrate buffer, pH 5.0 with 0.4 mg OPD per ml and 0.2 mg urea peroxide per ml. After incubation in the dark at room temperature for 60 min, the enzyme colour reaction was stopped by adding 0.05 ml 4 N sulphuric acid.

ELISA

The double antibody sandwich assay for the detection of rotavirus antigens was performed as described elsewhere (Ellens et al., 1978). One hundred μl volumes of a standard rotavirus suspension were diluted in 2-fold steps in polystyrene microtitre plates coated with bovine antibody against rotavirus. After incubation for 3 h at $37^{\circ}C$, the plates were washed and in- cubated with anti-rotavirus conjugate for 1 h at $37^{\circ}C$. A further washing was followed by the addition of the substrate solution. Absorption values of the reaction product were measured at 474 nm in a colorimeter equipped with a 80 μl flush cell. Before measuring, the trays were shaken for 2 min; samples with an A474 of more than 2 were diluted with an equal volume of water. P/N values were expressed as the ratio of the extinction values of the test sample and the negative control (i.e. PBS instead of rotavirus antigen).

RESULTS

A solution of commercially available 5-AS (1 mg/ml) in demineralised water, brought to a pH of 6.0 and containing hydrogen peroxide (conventio- nal 5-AS substrate solution), is slightly coloured with an A474 of approx- imately 0.1. On standing at room temperature, the colour intensity in- creases by about 0.08 A474 units per h. A coloured blank, especially when its colour intensity increases with time, will result in low P/N values for positive test samples.

Therefore we started to purify 5-AS by recrystallisation in the pre- sence of sodium bisulphite to prevent further oxidation of 5-AS. The puri- fied product was dissolved in phosphate buffer containing EDTA, followed by the addition of hydrogen peroxide (modified 5-AS substrate solution). A phosphate buffer containing EDTA was chosen to control the pH during the enzymatic reaction and to bind bivalent cations.

The modified substrate solution showed almost negligible optical dens- ity at all 5-AS concentrations tested (0.5-2.0 mg/ml). The A474 values were considerably lower than those for the conventional substrate solutions, employing the same 5-AS concentrations. In addition, the absorption values of modified substrate solutions hardly increased upon storage at room temp- erature (less than 0.005 A474 units per h).

The usefulness of modified substrate solutions was investigated in the ELISA for the detection of rotavirus antigens. In this experiment we com- pared A474 and P/N values measured with conventional and modified sub- strate solutions containing varying concentrations of 5-AS (Fig. 1). The ELISA was performed using a 1:200 dilution of standard rotavirus anti- gen. The results demonstrate that with both substrate solutions the absorp- tion values increased with higher 5-AS concentrations. However, for each concentration of 5-AS tested, higher absorption values were obtained with the modified substrate solutions than with the conventional ones. In contrast, the A474 of the PBS controls were considerably lower when the modified substrate solutions were used (Fig. 1). Expression of these data as P/N values showed that the use of the modified substrate solutions led to P/N values at least 5 times higher than those calculated from experiments with the conventional 5-AS solutions. Moreover, in the modified system the P/N values remained constant for 5-AS concentrations between 0.5 and 3.0 mg/ml, whereas in the conventional system increasing substrate concentrations led to decreasing P/N values (Fig. 1). Because of the limited solubility of the crude 5-AS in water, concentrations of over 2 mg/ml could not be tested.

In another experiment P/N values were determined at different times after addition of the conventional or the modified substrate solution to the test system. Both solutions contained 1 mg of 5-AS per ml. In each instance the P/N value obtained with the modified substrate solution was higher than that obtained with the conventional one (not shown). After addition of the modified substrate solution increasing P/N values were found for 2-3 h. Then the P/N values reached a plateau and remained constant even after overnight incubation. In contrast, P/N values obtained with the conventional substrate solution were maximal within 1 h of incubation and decreased rapidly thereafter.

Finally, we were able to demonstrate that an 8-fold increase in the sensitivity of the ELISA for the detection of rotavirus antigen was ob-

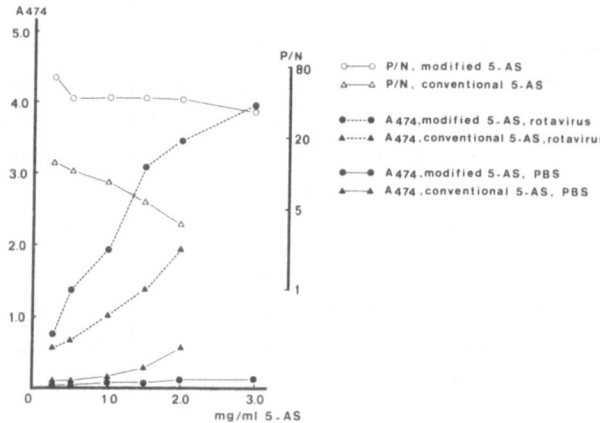

Fig. 1. ELISA A474 and P/N values obtained with conventional and modified substrate solutions containing different concentrations of 5-AS. A 1:200 dilution of standard rotavirus antigen was used. Absorption values were measured 2 h after addition of the substrate solution.

tained when antigen titers were determined with the modified substrate solution instead of the conventional one (not shown).

Since it is assumed that OPD is one of the most sensitive peroxidase substrates in enzyme immunoassays, we then compared the sensitivity of the rotavirus ELISA employing both OPD and the modified 5-AS solution. The absorption values obtained with OPD were higher than those obtained with 5-AS both after 1 h and after 18 h of incubation at room temperature. However, this did not result in higher P/N values because of the 3.8-fold higher value of the OPD blank as compared with the 5-AS blank (Fig. 2).

DISCUSSION

Using conventional 5-AS substrate solutions, optimal P/N values were obtained when low concentrations of 5-AS and short incubation times were used. The A474 values obtained under these conditions were low and visual reading was difficult due to coloured blanks. In addition, because the P/N values are influenced by the time of incubation and since it is impossible to stop the reaction completely (Bullock and Walls, 1977), each test must be read after a pre-set time. However, when modified 5-AS substrate solutions were used, neither the 5-AS concentration nor the in-

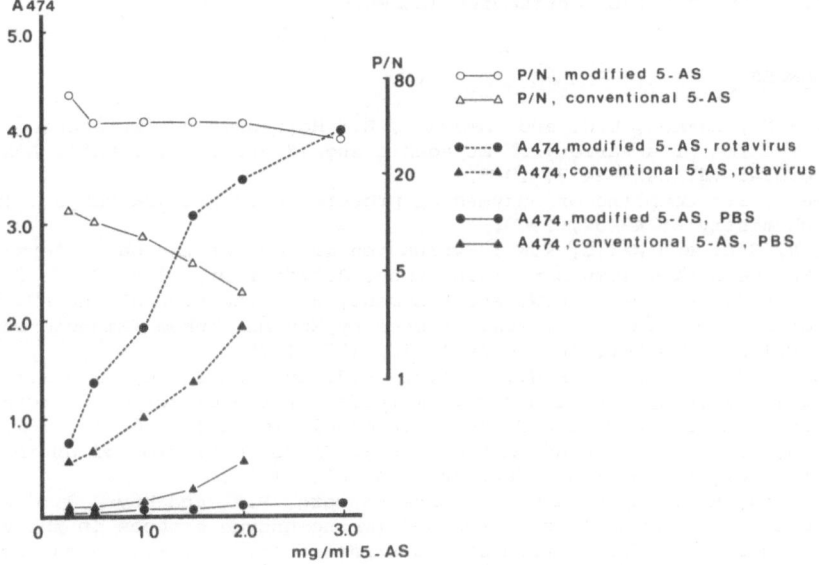

Fig. 2. Comparison of OPD and 5-AS as peroxidase substrates in the ELISA for the detection of rotavirus. A: A474 values; the blanks with the modified 5-AS substrate solution (PBS instead of rotavirus) measured 0.07 and 0.08 after 1 and 18 h, respectively and the blank with the OPD substrate solution measured 0.27 after 1 h. B: P/N values.

cubation time greatly influenced the P/N values obtained. Thus, at 5-AS
concentrations normally used in ELISA, the test can be read at any time
between 2 and 18 h after addition of the substrate. The plates can even
be stored for several days at 4°C, or for weeks at -20°C without signif-
cant loss of information. Besides, the low blank values with the modified
substrate solution facilitate visual reading of the plates.

The P/N values obtained with the modified 5-AS substrate solution were
at least 4-fold higher than those obtained with conventional 5-AS, independent of the substrate concentration and of the incubation time used. These
higher P/N values led to an 8-fold increase in the sensitivity of the rota-
virus-ELISA.

No significant difference in sensitivity for the detection of rotavirus antigens could be demonstrated between the ELISA carried out with the
modified 5-AS substrate or with OPD (Fig. 2). However, since special care
is needed in handling OPD because of its photosensitive and mutagenic properties (Ames et al., 1975; Voller et al., 1979), whereas with 5-AS no
mutagenic action was observed (Voogd et al., 1980), we prefer the use of
the modified 5-AS solution for routine ELISAs to detect antigens (Ellens
et al., 1978; 1979) or antibodies (Houwers and Gielkens 1979).

REFERENCES

Ames, B.N., Kammen, H.O. and Yamasaki, E.: Hair dyes are mutagenic: identi-
    fication of a variety of mutagenic ingredients. Proc. Natl. Acad. Sci.
    U.S.A. 72: 2423-2427, 1975.
Avrameas, S.: Coupling of enzymes to proteins with glutaraldehyde. Immuno-
    chemistry 6: 43-52, 1969.
Bullock, S.L. and Walls, K.W.: Evaluation of some of the parameters of the
    Enzyme-linked Immunospecific Assay. J.Infect.Dis. 136: S 279-285, 1977.
Ellens, D.J., De Leeuw, P.W. and Rozemond, H.: Detection of the K99 antigen
    of *Escherichia coli* in calf faeces by Enzyme-linked Immunosorbent Assay
    (ELISA). The Vet. Quarterly 1: 169-175, 1979.
Ellens, D.J., De Leeuw, P.W., Straver, P.J. and Van Balken, J.A.M.:
    Comparison of five diagnostic methods for the detection of rotavirus
    antigens in calf faeces. Med. Microbiol. Immunol. 166: 157-163, 1978.
Houwers, D.J. and Gielkens, A.L.J.: An ELISA for detection of antibodies
    to maedi/visna virus. Vet.Rec. 104: 611, 1979.
Ruitenberg, E.J., Ljungstrom, I., Steerenberg, P.A. and Buys, J.: Appli-
    cation of immunofluorescence and immuno-enzyme methods in the sero-
    diagnosis of *Trichinella spiralis* infection. Ann. N.Y. Acad. Sci.
    254: 296-303, 1975.
Voller, A., Bidwell, D.E. and Bartlett, A.: The Enzyme-linked Immunosorbent
    Assay (ELISA), 1979, (Dynatech. Europe, Guernsey).
Voogd, C.E., Van Der Stel, J.J. and Jacobs, J.J.J.A.A.: On the mutagenic
    action of some enzyme immunoassay substrates. J. Immunol. methods 36:
    55-61, 1980.

Wolters, G., Kuipers, L., Kacaki, J. and Schuurs, A.: Solid phase enzyme-
immunoassay for detection of hepatitis B surface antigen. J. Clin.
Pathol. 39: 873-879, 1976.

ELISA FOR THE DETECTION OF ROTAVIRUS AND
ROTAVIRUS/ANTIBODY COMPLEXES IN FAECES

R. Scherrer [1], G. Corthier [2], R. L'Haridon [3]

(1) Station de Virologie et d'Immunologie, INRA ,
78850 - Thiverval-Grignon France

(2) Laboratoire de Pathologie Porcine, INRA,
78850- Thiverval-Grignon, France

(3) Laboratoire de Pathologie du Bétail et des
Animaux de Basse-Cour, ENV, 94701 Maisons-Alfort
France.

ABSTRACT

A direct microplate ELISA for the detection and quantitation of bovine rotavirus is described. The assay permitted the detection of less than 5 ng virus/ml in purified preparations and in faecal samples, providing that the samples contained enough virus so that the assay could be performed at dilutions $\geq 1:1000$. In spite of a reduction in the sensitivity of the test at high concentrations of faecal material, the direct assay proved, in practice, to be more efficient than was electron microscopy. Results on the excretion of rotavirus in the course of infections and on the incidence of rotavirus infections among calves and older animals are presented and discussed.

A variant procedure that permits the detection of rotavirus immune complexes is described. Preliminar results are presented indicating that this test may constitute a useful tool in diagnostic work and in immunological investigations.

INTRODUCTION

The first microplate ELISA that was developed in order to detect rotavirus in faeces (Scherrer and Bernard 1977) was a non competitive double-sandwich method involving the use of a rabbit anti rotavirus serum to precoat the wells ; antigens, trapped on the sensitized solid phase were detected by the addition of an anti rotavirus bovine serum followed by addition of an anti bovine-Ig conjugate and assay of the enzyme reaction with its substrate. Later on, the technique was simplified so that the virus could be detected directly with an anti rotavirus conjugate. This report describes briefly some characteristics of the direct assay together with results obtained with this test in diagnostic

work and epidemiological investigations. A variant procedure that permits
the detection of rotavirus immune complexes will also be described.

MATERIALS AND METHODS

1. ELISA for the detection and quantitation of bovine rotavirus in faeces.

Anti-rotavirus sera were produced in seronegative rabbits or goats.
Animals were inoculated intramuscularly with purified calf rotavirus (cell
culture adapted Thiverval strain) (L'Haridon and Scherrer, 1976) in complete Freund's adjuvant. Four to five weeks later, the animals were rein-
jected intraveneously with purified virus alone and bled six to eight days
after the second injection (titres of standard rabbit and goat antisera
were respectively 20,000 and 35,000 by indirect immunofluorescent test on
preinfected cell-cultures). After precipitation of one volume serum with
Na_2SO_4 (36 % and 34 %) the globulin fraction was redissolved in one
volume phosphate-buffered saline (PBS) pH 7.4, and small aliquots stored
at − 80°C until use. The antirotavirus conjugate used throughout this
study was obtained by coupling the Ig fraction of rabbit anti rotavirus
serum with alkaline phosphatase according to the technique described by
Engvall and Perlmann, 1972.

The assays were performed in polystyrene microplates (Linbro réf.
IS-FB-90 ; Flow laboratories) using a non competitive sandwich method.
Coating of the wells involved an overnight incubation at 20°C with a
1/7000 dilution of the anti rotavirus Ig fraction (goat) in carbonate
buffer pH 9.6. Incubation with test samples, diluted in PBS-Tween 0.05 %
was for two hours at 20°C and incubation with the conjugate (diluted
1:37,000 in PBS-Tween 0.05 % for 2.5 h at 20°C).The substrate (p-nitrophenylphosphate 1 mg/ml in diethanolamine buffer pH 9.8) was reacted for
60 minutes at 37°C. Absorbancy was measured at 405 nm in the Titertek[R]
Multiskan ELISA reader.

2. ELISA for the detection of rotavirus immune-complexes.

The technique was applied to the detection of rotavirus/antibody
complexes in the faeces of pigs and involved the following steps :
sensitization of plates with an anti rotavirus IgG preparation produced
in a rabbit (3 hours at 37°C) - incubation with serially diluted faecal
extracts (overnight at 20°C) - incubation for 3 hours at 37°C with an
anti pig-Ig (L chain) conjugate (alkaline phosphatase) and finally, incubation with the substrate solution as above. The anti rotavirus serum was

obtained after three intramuscular injections with purified pig rotavirus
in complete Freund's adjuvant. The serum was precipitated with ammonium
sulfate (50 %) and the IgG purified by ion exchange on a DEAE Sephadex
column. The anti pig-Ig serum was obtained by hyperimmunization of a rabbit with pure pig IgG (Harboe and Ingild, 1973). The antiserum was then
absorbed with pure pig IgM, insolubilized with glutaraldehyde (Avrameas,
1969) and anti L chain antibodies eluted at pH 2.8. Coupling with alkaline phosphatase was performed according to the technique described by
Avrameas 1969.

RESULTS

1. Sensitivity of ELISA for the detection of bovine rotavirus in purified
   preparations and in faeces.

When purified rotavirus particles were used in the standard assay,
typical dose-response curves were obtained and it was shown that the
technique allows the detection of less than 10 ng double-shelled particles
per ml and less than 5 ng single-shelled particles per ml (fig. 1 and 2).
This range of sensitivity may correspond to about 10^7 to 5×10^7 particles
per ml. Thus, the sensitivity of the assay lies close to that offered by a
careful examination in the electron microscope, as far as the detection
of virions is concerned.

When relative high amounts of purified particles were introduced into
negative faeces and the mixture serially diluted, the sensitivity of the
assay was similar to that involving purified virus alone. However, it was
noticed that the sensitivity of the test, for detecting small amounts of
virus in undiluted faeces, or even in low dilutions of faeces, was lowered
as shown in fig. 3.

When the test was applied to samples collected from naturally-infec-
ted or experimentally-infected calves, curves very similar to that seen
in fig 1 or 2 were often obtained (fig. 4, curve A). Some specimens however,
gave a curve exhibiting a significant drop of the A 405 values (fig. 4,
curve B) at the lowest dilutions of faeces. This effect did not appear to
be correlated with the presence of antigen in excess but rather with the
presence of faecal material at high concentrations.

To compare the relative sensitivities of the direct ELISA and electron microscopy (EM) (negative staining of the supernatants of faeces
diluted 1:3) in routine diagnostic work, a total of 163 faecal samples
from healthy and diarrhoeic calves, were tested using both techniques.

As shown in table I, all samples scored positif by E M , except one, were positive by ELISA. In case of samples scored negative by EM, 9 out of 99 appeared weakly positive by ELISA. However, after ultracentrifugation of these 9 specimens and reexamination by EM, it came out that 5 did contain a few identifiable particles ; furthermore, the presence of rotaviral antigens could be confirmed in an additional sample by a blocking test using an anti rotavirus bovine serum. Finally, three samples remained doubtful and could be considered eventually as false positive reactions.

2. Use of ELISA in the study of rotaviral infections and in epidemiological investigations.

Figure 5 and 6 are to show that ELISA constitutes a well-suited technique to follow quantitatively the excretion of rotavirus in the course of infections and to assess the role of the virus in the disease. Fig. 5 illustrates a typical example of an experimentally-induced rotaviral diarrhoea in a calf. As can be noted here there is a strict concomitance between the onset of the disease and the appearance of high amounts of virus in the faeces. Furthermore, one also notices a nice correlation between the duration of diarrhoea and the duration of intense shedding of the virus. In field studies a number of cases of diarrhoea were also shown to correlate stricktly with an episode of viral excretion, as shown in fig. 6. Of course, diarrhoeic episodes not associated with rotavirus, as well as asymptomatic infections were also observed.

In order to evaluate the incidence of rotavirus infections, a survey was conducted by the Laboratory in three different herds in 1978/1979 and 1979/1980 on healthy and diarrhoeic calves one to twenty days old, as well as on cows and dams at the time of parturition. A total of 164 specimens collected from 77 calves were analysed by ELISA (table II). It was shown that the rotavirus was associated with 37 cases of diarrhoea out of 48 (77 %). In contrast, the virus was found in 7 specimens only out of 97 samples collected dayly from 10 healthy calves and in one calf only out of 19 healthy calves.

In the same herds a total of 60 faecal samples, collected from dams at the time of parturition and a total of 20 other specimens from cows were analyzed for the presence of rotavirus. As shown in table II, all these specimens were negative.

3. ELISA for the detection of rotavirus immune complexes.

The technique (see materials and methods) was applied to the detection of immune complexes in the faeces of pigs. To estimate the reliability of the test the later was applied, together with the direct ELISA (detection of antigens alone) to artificial mixtures of a purified pig rotavirus suspension with serial dilutions of an anti pig rotavirus serum (fig. 7). At high concentrations of antiserum neither immune complexes (I.C.) nor rotavirus could be detected, probably as a consequence of complete saturation of rotavirus antigens by specific antibodies. Inside a range of intermediate serum dilutions both immune complexes and rotavirus were detectable : however, there was also a narrow dilution range where the I.C. test appeared significantly positive while the direct ELISA appeared negative or nearly so. At high serum dilutions little or no I.C. were found and correlatively the rotavirus particles became fully detectable.

Using both tests, a total of 62 faecal samples (23 diarrhoeic and 39 normal) were tested for the presence of rotavirus and I.C. Positive and negative samples by both tests were respectively 9 and 41. Rotavirus alone was detected in 6 samples and I.C. alone in 6 other samples.

CONCLUSION

The results reported here indicate that the sensitivity of the direct ELISA, for detecting rotavirus in faeces, is at least as high or even higher in practice, than that offered by an examination of ultracentrifuged specimens in the electron microscope. Thus, considering the simplicity of the direct assay and the fact that quantitative data can be obtained, it makes no doubt that it is one of the most practical method for diagnosis and epidemiological studies. Yet, one must also keep in mind that problems may arise when small amounts of particles and/or antigens are to be found in undiluted faeces. Occasionally, false negative results may be obtained : the later are best explained when antibodies are present in the intestinal tract, but other factors, that may lower the sensitivity of the assay and which appear to be directly related to a high concentration of faecal material, must also be considered. The preliminar results obtained with the ELISA adapted to the detection of I.C., indicate that this assay not only constitutes a useful tool for studying several aspects of intestinal immunity but it may also be of value for detecting the presence of rotavirus under conditions where the direct assay yields doubtful or unsatisfactory results. In any case, weak positive results should be confirmed either by electron microscopic techniques or by ELISA using a blocking serum.

Using the direct ELISA to estimate the incidence of rotavirus infections among calves, we were able to confirm and extend earlier observations (Scherrer et al. 1976) made by electron microscopy. The fact that the rotavirus was clearly found in a high percentage of diarrhoeic calves and only in a low percentage of healthy calves, evidences the aetiological role this virus must play in the disease. None of the 80 samples collected from cows and dams were shown to be positif for rotavirus. This confirms the general agreement on the weak susceptibility of older animals to rotavirus infections. However, this does not necessarily mean that reinfections do not occur, but if they occur, it is likely that in most cases the virus multiplies to such a low degree that it will not be detectable in the faeces.

ACKNOWLEDGMENTS
This work was supported in part by a DGRST contract n° 77.7.1850. We thank Chantal Feynerol and Nathalie Melik for technical assistance and M. Daburon and M. Vicaire for supplying the field specimens.

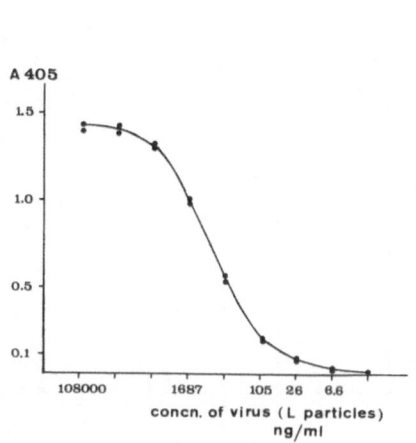

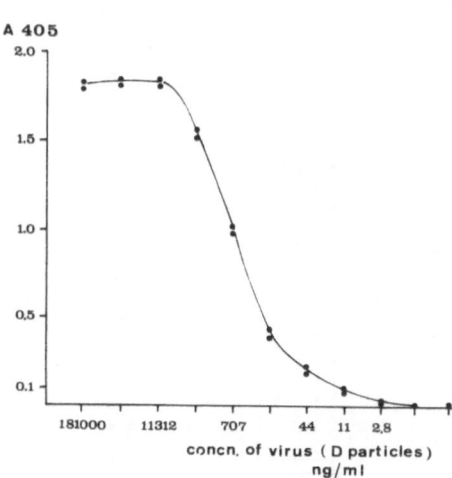

Fig. 1 : Dose-response curve for double shelled bovine rotavirus particles. The virus was purified according to the technique described by Cohen, 1977. The concentration of particles was estimated from the relationship established for reovirus : 9.1. A 260 nm = 1 mg/ml (Farrell et al. 1974)

Fig. 2 : Dose-response curve for single-shelled rotavirus particles.

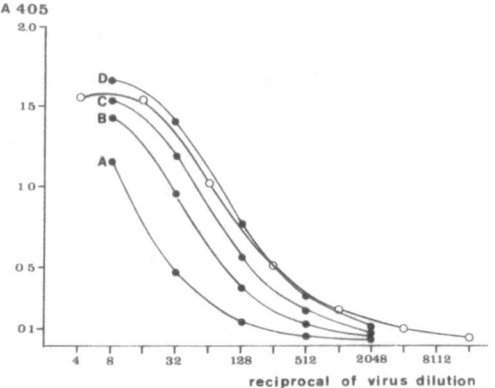

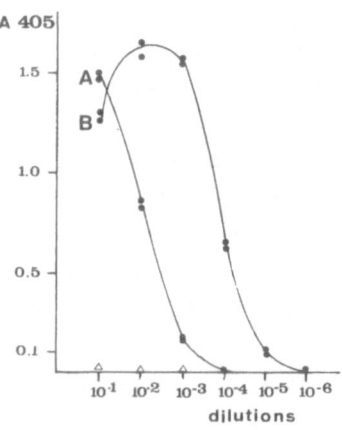

Fig. 3 : Dose-response curves for purified
rotavirus particles (single and double-
shelled) in presence of faeces.
O——O Reference dose-response curve (purified virus alone). Curves A, B, C and D
were obtained by diluting the virus in a
negative faecal extract.(A): dilution of the
faecal extract 1:10 constant. (B) : 1:50
constant (C) : 1:100 constant (D):1:1000
constant.

Fig. 4 : Typical ELISA curves obtained with faecal
samples collected from rotavirus infected calves.
Notice the drop of the
A 405 values at the lowest
dilutions of sample B.

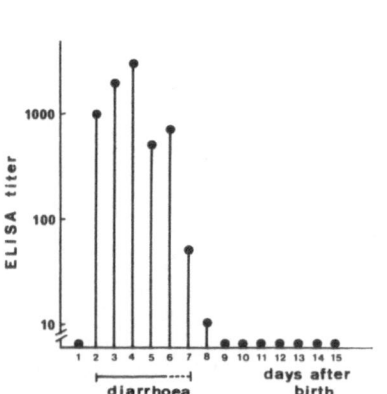

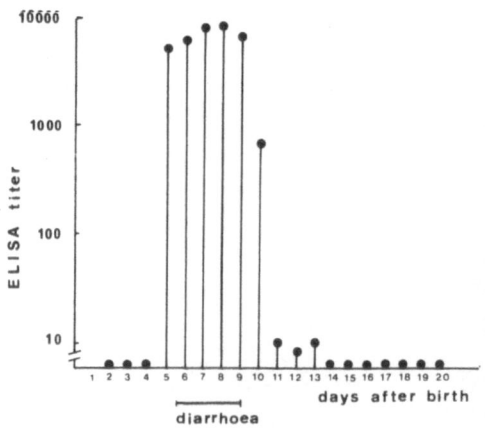

Fig. 5 : Excretion of virus in the
course of an experimentally-induced
rotaviral diarrhea. The relative
ELISA titres are expressed as the
reciprocal of the sample dilution
corresponding to an A 405 of 0.2
in the standard assay.

Fig. 6 : Excretion of rotavirus in
the course of a natural case of
diarrhea.

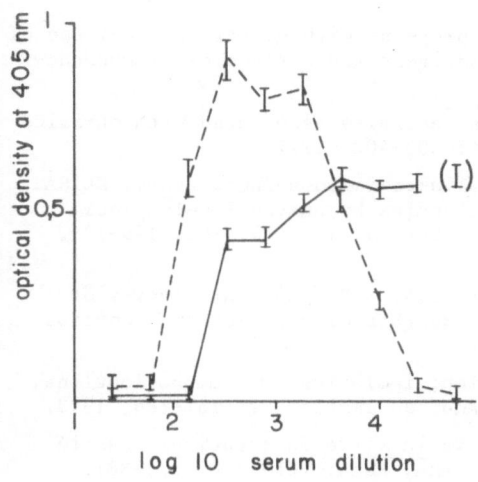

Fig. 7 : Detection of rotavirus/
antibody complexes in artificial
mixtures of a purified pig rotavirus suspension with serial
dilutions of an anti pig-rotavi-
rus serum.
⊢--⊣detection of immune complexes
as a function of antiserum concentration
⊢——⊣detection of rotavirus antigens by the direct ELISA.

TABLE I - DETECTION OF ROTAVIRUS ANTIGENS IN FAECES BY E.M. AND ELISA

E . M .		ELISA	
Positive samples		Positive	Negative
64		63	1
Negative samples		Positive	Negative
99		9	90

TABLE II - ROTAVIRUS INFECTIONS IN CALVES AND ADULTS

	SAMPLING	NUMBER OF SAMPLES	POSITIVE SAMPLES (ROTA)
DIARRHEIC CALVES	One sample on the 2nd day of disease	48	37
HEALTHY CALVES	every day	97 (from 10 calves)	7 (from 2 calves)
	the 6th day after birth	19	1
COWS	During a three month period after calving	20	0
DAMS	At the time of parturition	60	0

REFERENCES

Avrameas, S. : Coupling of enzymes to proteins with glutaraldehyde. Use of conjugates for the detection of antigens and antibodies. Immunochemistry 6: 43–52, 1969.

Cohen, J. : Ribonucleic acid polymerase activity associated with purified calf rotavirus. J. Gen. Virol. 36: 395–402, 1977.

Engvall, E. and Perlmann, P. : Enzyme linked immunosorbent assay, ELISA. III – Quantitation of specific antibodies by enzyme-labeled anti immunoglobulin in antigen-coated tubes. J. Immunol. 109: 129–135, 1972.

Farrel, J.A., Harvey, J.D. and Bellamy, A.R. : Biophysical studies of reovirus type 3. I – The molecular weights of reovirus and reovirus cores. Virology 62: 145–153, 1974.

Harboe, N. and Ingild, A. : Immunisation, isolation of immunoglobulins, estimation of antibody titer. Scand. J. Immunol. 2: 161–164, 1973.

L'Haridon, R. and Scherrer, R. : Culture in vitro du rotavirus associé aux diarrhées néonatales du veau. Ann. Rech. Vétér. 7: 373–381, 1976.

Scherrer, R. and Bernard, S. : Application d'une technique immunoenzymologique (ELISA) à la détection du rotavirus bovin et des anticorps dirigés contre lui. Ann. Microbiol. (Institut Pasteur) 128 A: 499–510, 1977.

Scherrer, R., Cohen, J., L'Haridon, R., Feynerol, C. and Fayet, J.C. : Reovirus-like agent (rotavirus) associated with neonatal calf gastroenteritis in France. Ann. Rech. Vétér. 7: 25–31, 1976.

RNA GEL ELECTROPHORESIS: A TECHNIQUE TO MONITOR LABORATORY CROSS-
CONTAMINATIONS AND GENETIC REASSORTMENT AMONGST ROTAVIRUS ISOLATES

S. Tzipori and M. Smith

Attwood Veterinary Research Laboratory, Westmeadows, Melbourne, 3047,

Australia.

ABSTRACT

The RNA of 2 isolates of simian rotavirus SA11 and another cell
culture adapted isolate 325, are compared using polyacrylamide slab gel
electrophoresis.   The 2 SA11 isolates differ in the positions of RNA
segments 3, 325 is believed to exist as a mixed population on the basis
of RNA analysis and the RNA pattern of the predominant viral element is
indistinguishable from that of one of the SA11 isolates.   It is
suggested that genetic reassortment of the RNA segments in mixed
infections can produce a progeny rotavirus with an altered genome.

INTRODUCTION

The number of rotavirus strains adapted to propagate in cell culture
is small.   These strains are used extensively for diagnosis, serological
survey, research and production of experimental vaccines in a large
number of laboratories across the world.   Recently the use of trypsin
has enhanced in vitro propagation of other rotavirus isolates.
Biochemical analysis of rotaviruses has revealed that the genome is
double stranded RNA and exists as at least 11 segments.   Gel electrophoresis, in the absence of routine cultivation and serotyping, has
become a useful technique for identification of different isolates and to
monitor their purity.

MATERIALS AND METHODS

The rotavirus SA11 was imported into Australia in 1977, and was
distributed to 2 laboratories in Melbourne.   Two years later, the RNA
electrophoretic profile of the SA11 propagated in the 2 separate
laboratories, was examined.

The rotavirus 325 was derived from a human rotavirus isolate
(500) that was serially passaged 5 times in young dogs (Tzipori and
Makin, 1978).   An attempt was made to adapt this rotavirus to grow in
monkey (SK) cell culture and after approximately 10 subcultures the RNA
of this isolate 325 was analysed.   Further 6 rapid subcultures of 325

was carried out in 2 separate cultures, in SK primary cells and in the
MA104 cell line.   The RNAS of 325 harvested from SK and MA104, were
analysed.

Extracted rotavirus RNA (Smith and Tzipori, 1979) was subjected to
electrophoresis in a 10% polyacrylamide gel with a discontinuous buffer
system (Laemmli, 1970) for 4.5 hours at 40 mA at room temperature.   The
gel was stained with ethidium bromide for half one hour.

RESULTS

The RNA gel electrophoresis of the 2 SA11 (known as A and M) which
originated from the same stock preparations of simian rotavirus, showed
that segment 3 of A is of slightly higher molecular weight than the
corresponding segment in M.   Co-electrophoresis of SA11 A and SA11 M
confirmed these variations.

There appeared to be at least 2 different electrophoretic types
present in 325 (13 segments) with predominantly one type of rotavirus
RNA (SA11 M) and a contaminating virus present in lower quantities.
Attempts have been made to elucidate the origin of the minor
contaminating RNA.   Co-electrophoresis of 325 with the rotavirus of
human origin (500) from which it was derived, indicated that the 2 less
intensely staining RNA bands (segments 1 and 3) of higher molecular
weights had come from this source.

Six additional passages of 325 in SK cells did not alter the pattern
of the 13 segment profile.   Propagation in MA104 on the other hand
seems to have eliminated the minor contaminating components and the profile
was restored back to 11 segments consistent with that of SA11M.

DISCUSSION

The RNA migration pattern of rotavirus is reportedly a stable
characteristic and the CODY strain of calf rotavirus has maintained
a stable genome for over 200 passages in vitro and in vivo (Kalika et al.,
1978).   During co-infection of cells in culture with SA11M and
unidentified contaminating unadapted rotavirus, genetic reassortment may
have occurred and the new emerging electrophoretic type (SA11A) had
its 3rd segment replaced with one of higher molecular weight.   Genetic
reassortment has been reported for the other 2 members of the
REOVIRIDAE group, the ORBIVIRUSES (Gorman et al., 1974) and the
REOVIRUSES (Joklik, 1974).   Presumably both the original SA11M and

SA11A with the newly replaced 3rd segment must have co-existed in cell culture at some time, until SA11A predominated over the 2 years period.

It is apparent that 325 became contaminated with the cell culture adapted SA11M and now it appears to contain a mixture of at least 2 co-existing electrophoretic types in SK cells, one being the predominant SA11M and the second is SA11M that had its 1st and 3rd segments replaced. The 2 newly acquired segments must have originated from the rotavirus of human origin (500). The 2 electrophoretic types were eventually resolved into one (SA11M) by 6 serial subcultures in MA104 cell line but not in SK primary cells.

If gene reassortment readily occurs between rotaviruses _in vitro_ then a similar process may operate _in vivo_. Large numbers of interspecies and intraspecies electrophoretic types have now been reported. Simultaneous infection with different rotavirus isolates and subsequent gene reassortment, could be responsible for the vast numbers of existing variations. There is evidence that experimental co-infection of animals can also lead to genetic reassortment (Tzipori and Smith, unpublished data).

Contaminations of cell culture adapted rotaviruses with wild types or vice versa leading to genetic reassortment appear to occur readily and RNA gel electrophoresis is the most sensitive technique to detect it.

REFERENCES

Gorman, B.M., Taylor, J., Walker, P.J. and Young P.R.: The isolation of recombinants between related orbiviruses. J. Gen. Virol. 41: 333-342, 1978.

Joklik, W.K.: Reproduction of reoviridae. In: Fraenkel-Conrat, H., Wagner, R.R. - Comprehensive Virology 2: 231-334, 1974.

Kalika, A.R., Sereno, M.M. Wyatt, R.G., Mebus, C.A., Chanock, R.M. and Kapikian, A.Z.: Comparison of human and animal rotavirus strains by gel electrophoresis of viral RNA. Virol. 87: 247-255, 1978.

Laemmli, U.K.: Cleavage of structural proteins during assembly of the head of bacteriophage T4. Nature 227: 680-685, 1970.

Smith, M. and Tzipori, S.: Gel electrophoresis of rotavirus RNA derived from 6 different animal species. Aust. J. Biol. Med. Sc. 57: 583-585, 1979.

Tzipori, S. and Makin, T.: Propagation of human rotavirus in young dogs.
     Vet. Microbiol. 3:   55-63, 1978.

THE NEUTRALISATION OF THE INDIRECT IMMUNOFLUORESCENCE TEST AND
THE IMMUNODIFFUSION TEST : TWO DETECTION METHODS FOR NEONATAL
CALF DIARRHOEA VIRUSES.
A COMPARATIVE STUDY WITH ELISA AND ELECTRON MICROSCOPY

E. Van Opdenbosch and Wellemans G.
Nationaal Instituut voor Diergeneeskundig Onderzoek
Groeselenberg 99 - 1180 Brussel (Belgium)
and
D.J. Ellens and De Leeuw P.W.
Centraal Diergeneeskundig Instituut
Houtribweg 39 - 8221 RA Lelystad (The Netherlands)

ABSTRACT

A comparative study of the neutralisation of the indirect immunofluorescence (NIIF) test, the immunodiffusion (ID) tes, enzyme-linked
immunosorbent assay (ELISA) and electron microscopy (EM) for the detection
of rotaviruses in calf faeces was done at the Nationaal Instituut voor
Diergeneeskundig Onderzoek (NIDO) in Belgium and the Centraal Diergeneeskundig Instituut (CDI) in The Netherlands. A total of 93 faecal samples was
examined. Sixty-two per cent was positive for rotavirus by EM, 59 % with
the NIIF test, 58 % with the ID test and 57 % with ELISA. All samples negative by EM were also negative in the NIIF and the ID test but three of these
samples were found positive in the ELISA.

Forty-three faecal samples were tested for the presence of bovine
coronavirus. Eleven samples were scored positive by EM of which ten were
positive in the NIIF test and five in ELISA. Two other samples were found
positive by ELISA only.

INTRODUCTION

In recent years several new methods have been developed for the detection of enteric viruses in faecal material, f.e. enzyme-linked immunosorbent assay (ELISA) (1, 3, 4), the neutralisation of the indirect immunofluorescence (NIIF) test (6) and an immunodiffusion (ID) test (5). To
compare the results of these methods with each other and with those of electron microscopy (EM), a comparative study was undertaken in which the
Nationaal Instituut voor Diergeneeskundig Onderzoek (NIDO) in Belgium and
the Centraal Diergeneeskundig Instituut (CDI) in The Netherlands partici-
pated.

MATERIAL AND METHODS

Faecal samples

The faecal samples used in this study originated from diarrhoeic as well as healthy calves. The majority of the samples had been tested previously in one of the participating laboratories, i.e. they had been frozen twice at −20° C (before and after testing) before they were sent to the other laboratory.

A total of 93 samples was examined for the presence of rotaviruses in the NIIF test, the ID test and by EM in the NIDO, and by EM and ELISA in the CDI. In addition, 43 samples were examined for the presence of bovine coronaviruses in the NIIF test and by EM in the NIDO and by ELISA in the CDI.

Virus detection methods

The ELISA's for the detection of rotavirus and bovine coronaviruses in faecal samples have been described (1, 3). Further details can be found in the rotavirus manual of the Central Veterinary Institute, The Netherlands, in these proceedings.

The NIIF test and the ID test have also been described (6, 5); laboratory manuals of both tests are included in these proceedings.

Electron microscopy was performed as follows. In the NIDO faecal material was diluted 2:3 in PBS, mixed with an ultraturrax, and centrifuged at 3,000 rpm for 15 min. The supernatant was applied to carbon-coated grids and strained with a solution of 2 % uranyl acetate. The grids were examined for 15 min using a Philips TEM201 electron microscope. In the CDI faecal extracts were applied to carbon-coated grids and stained with a solution of 2 % PTA adjusted to pH 6.2 with KOH. Ten squares of a 400-mesh grid were examined for the presence of rotavirus particles using a Jeol 100C electron microscope at a magnification of 50,000.

Each faecal sample was tested in two institutes; a sample is recorded rotavirus-positive if at least one of the examinations yielded positive results.

RESULTS

The results obtained with the different tests for the detection of rotavirus are shown on fig.1.

Fig. 1. Comparison of different tests for the detection of rotavirus in
faeces of calves

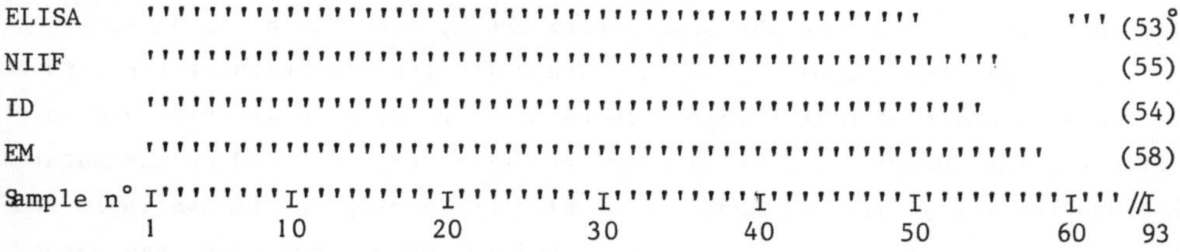

```
ELISA     '''''''''''''''''''''''''''''''''''''''''''''''''            ''' (53°)
NIIF      '''''''''''''''''''''''''''''''''''''''''''''''''''''''' ''''    (55)
ID        ''''''''''''''''''''''''''''''''''''''''''''''''''''''''''       (54)
EM        ''''''''''''''''''''''''''''''''''''''''''''''''''''''''''''''   (58)
Sample n° I'''''''''I'''''''''I'''''''''I'''''''''I'''''''''I'''''''''I'''//I
          1       10        20        30        40        50        60   93
```
° Total number of samples positive

Fifty-eight out of 93 faecal samples were scored positive by EM, 55 in
the NIIF test, 54 in the ID test and 53 by ELISA. Rotavirus antigens were
detected by all four tests in 50 samples and by three tests in four other
samples. With ELISA three samples were found positive that were negative in
the other tests.

Fig.2 shows the results of the different tests for the detection of
bovine coronaviruses. Eleven out of 43 samples were scored positive by EM;
ten in the NIIF test and seven by ELISA. Five samples were positive in all
three tests, ten samples in two samples were scored positive by ELISA only.

Fig.2 Comparison of different tests for the detection of bovine coronaviruses in faeces of calves.

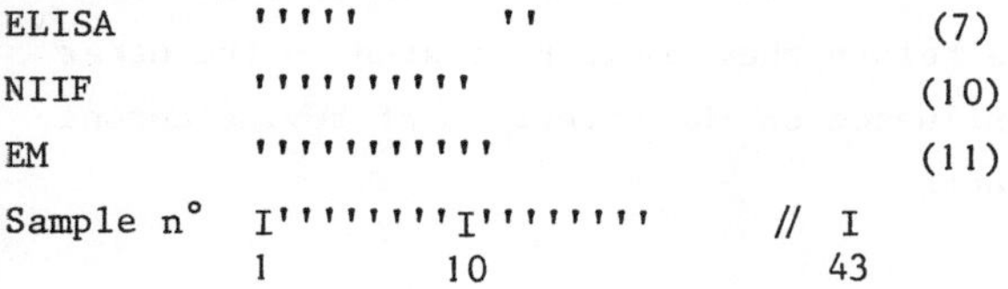

```
ELISA     '''''      ''                (7)
NIIF      '''''''''''                  (10)
EM        '''''''''''                  (11)
Sample n° I'''''''''I'''''''''    //  I
          1       10              43
```

CONCLUSIONS

The results of the four tests used in this study for the detection of
rotavirus in faecal samples corresponded rather well (Fig.1). The unex-
pectedly high EM score is undoubtedly influenced by the fact that each
sample was tested in two different laboratories and that the time spent on
each sample was unusually long. Furthermore, rotavirus-antibody complexes
present in faecal samples may prevent a positive diagnosis in the ELISA,
the NIIF and the ID test, whereas they are easily detected by EM (2). The
specificity of the NIIF and the ID test is demonstrated by the fact that all
samples found positive in these two tests were also scored positive by EM.

Whether the three faecal samples that reacted positively in the ELISA but
not in the other tests are indeed positive remains an open question, despite
the fact that they passed the specificity check, i.e. the blocking test.

Since all tests employed in this study for the detection of rotaviruses
in faecal samples of calves appear to be of comparable sensitivity and specificity, the choice for a particular laboratory may be based on the future
use and the local circumstances. If an electron microscope is available and
limited numbers of samples have to be examined, EM appears to be the method
of choice. The ID test is probably the most simple test of the four employed
here; neither expensive equipment nor tissue culture facilities are required.
The NIIF test has the advantage that it does not require mono-specific antisera. This may be of particular significance for laboratories that do not
have the disposal of gnotobiotic or SPF calves. The ELISA has the usual
advantages of this type of assay, i.e. the large numbers of samples that
can be handled and the speed with which the results become available. If
necessary the ELISA can be completed within the same day, whereas the ID
test takes 24 h and the NIIF test 36 h.

The results of the different tests used for the detection of bovine
coronaviruses (Fig.2) indicate that the NIIF test is nearly as sensitive
as (extensive) EM and slightly more sensitive than ELISA. However, as only
a limited number of samples tested were positive, definite conclusions
await futher work. In addition, the fact that the faecal samples had been
frozen and thawed at least twice before they could be tested in the other
laboratory, may have had more influence on the detection of bovine coronaviruses than on that of rotaviruses.

REFERENCES

1. Ellens, D.J., De Leeuw, P.W. : An enzyme linked immunosorbent assay
   (ELISA)for the diagnosis of rotavirus infections in calves. J.Clin.
   Microbiol. 6 : 530-532, 1977.
2. Ellens, D.J., De Leeuw, P.W., Straver, P.J. and Van Balken, J.A.M. : Comparison of five diagnostic methods for the detection of rotavirus antigens in calf faeces. Med.Microb.Immunol. 166 : 157-163, 1978.
3. Ellens, D.J., Van Balken, J.A.M. and De Leeuw, P.W. : Diagnosis of bovine
   coronavirus infections with hemadsorption-elution-hemagglutination
   assay (HEMA) and with enzyme-linked immunosorbent assay (ELISA).Proc.
   Second Int.Symp. on Neonatal Diarrhea, University of Saskatchewan,
   Canada, p.322-329, 1978.
4. Scherrer, B.S. : Application d'une technique immunoenzymologique (ELISA)
   à la détection du rotavirus bovin et des anticorps dirigés contre lui.
   Ann.Microbiol. (Institut Pasteur) 128A : 499-519, 1977.
5. Van Opdenbosch, E., Dekegel, D. and Wellemans, G. : De immunodiffusietest
   voor het opsporen van het Rotavirus in meststalen en darmfragmenten.

Vl.Dierg. Tijdschrift 47 : 276-291, 1978.
6. Wellemans, G., Van Opdenbosch, E., et Dekegel, D. : La neutralisation de l'immunofluorescence indirecte (NIFI) : une technique spécifique et quantitative pour la mise en évidence d'antigènes viraux. Ann.Med.Vét. 123 : 185-194, 1979.

COMPARISON OF DIAGNOSTIC PROCEDURES FOR BOVINE ROTAVIRUS

P.C. Grauballe, A. Meyling[*], B.F. Vestergaard and J. Genner

University of Copenhagen and State Veterinary Serumlaboratory[*]
Copenhagen, Denmark

Faecal samples or intestinal contents from 92 fatal cases of neonatal diarrhoea in calves were tested for rotavirus by the following methods. Electron microscopy (EM) was performed as previously described, by negative staining of bands obtained after centrifugation of clarified faecal suspensions on CsCl-gradients (Grauballe et al., 1977). Detection of fluorescent antigen by the use of FITC-conjugated rabbit anti bovine rotavirus antibodies (FA) was performed in two ways: either by direct staining of smears from intestinal contents or by staining of primary bovine kidney cells previously inoculated with the specimen as described (Meyling, 1974). Immunoelectro-osmophoresis (IEOP) and enzyme-linked immuno-sorbent assay (ELISA) were performed according to the manuals presented at this meeting, using the same antibodies for both assays, i.e. second generation polyspecific antibodies to human rotavirus prepared in rabbits by injection of immunoprecipitates as previously described (Grauballe et al., 1979).

In 30 specimens rotavirus was detected by all methods used, whereas in 51 specimens no rotavirus was detected by any of the methods. This means that the four methods used showed complete agreement in 81 of 92 cases, or in 88%. If all of the remaining 11 specimens in which rotavirus was detected by 1, 2 or 3 of the methods used are regarded as truly positive, the EM detected 73% (30/41), IEOP 76% (31/41), FA 83% (34/41) and ELISA 98% (40/41) of the specimens positive for rotavirus.

It is concluded that ELISA for bovine rotavirus, using a single antibody sandwich of rabbit antibody to human rotavirus as catching antibodies and the same antibodies conjugated to peroxydase as detecting antibodies, is a simple and sensitive method for diagnosis of rotavirus infections in calves.

The same reagents and test are used by others for detection of rotavirus in faecal samples from pigs with diarrhoea. At present it can be concluded that this method is suitable and reliable also for detection of porcine rotavirus as compared to EM and IEOP on the same specimens (Askaa, 1980).

REFERENCES

Askaa, J.: Personal communication, 1980.
Grauballe, P.C., Genner, J., Meyling, A. and Hornsleth, A.: Rapid Diagnosis of Rotavirus Infections: Comparison of Electron Microscopy and Immuno-electro-osmophoresis for the Detection of Rotavirus in Human Infantile Gastroenteritis. J. Gen. Virol. 35: 203-218, 1977.
Grauballe, P.C., Meyling A. and Genner, J.: Immunoelectrophoretic Studies of Rotaviruses: Preparation of Rabbit Antibodies to Immunoprecipitates of Human Rotavirus and Their Use for Identification of Specific and Common Antigens of Human and Bovine Rotavirus. In: Viral Enteritis, INSERM Symposia Series, Vol. 90, Ed. F. Bricout and R. Sherrer, pp. 413-427, 1979.
Meyling, A.: Reo-like Neonatal Calf Diarrhoea Virus Demonstrated in Denmark. Acta Vet. Scand. 15: 457-459, 1974.

THE DIAGNOSIS OF CORONAVIRUS-LIKE AGENT (CVLA) DIARRHEA

IN SUCKLING PIGS

P. Debouck, P. Callebaut and M. Pensaert

Laboratory of Virology, Faculty of Veterinary Medicine

University of Gent, Belgium

ABSTRACT

Two techniques are evaluated for the diagnosis of CVLA enteritis in suckling pigs. CVLA antigens can be demonstrated in the absorptive epithelial cells of the small intestine by the direct immunofluorescent staining test (IF). Very reliable results were obtained with this technique in piglets having diarrhea for only 3-4 days. Coronavirus particles can also be detected by electron microscopy (EM) in the feces of scouring pigs, but this should be followed by a specific identification test since there is no morphological difference between CVLA and transmissible gastroenteritis (TGE) virus. The EM is furthermore less sensitive than the IF test for the diagnosis of CVLA enteritis.

INTRODUCTION

The coronavirus-like agent (CVLA) has been described since 1977 as a pathogen for swine, causing enteritis in pigs of all ages (Pensaert, 1978; Debouck, 1980). The electron microscopical appearance of this virus indicates that it probably belongs to the Coronavirus family. The CVLA was also shown to be antigenically distinct from the 2 known porcine coronaviruses, Transmissible gastroenteritis (TGE) virus and Hemagglutinating encephalomyelitis virus. When a sudden outbreak of diarrhea occurs on a swine breeding farm, involving the piglets as well as the sows, then one should make a differential diagnosis between TGE and CVLA infection. This is very difficult to perform on the basis of the clinical signs. Up to now, it is impossible to grow the CVLA in tissue culture. The etiologic diagnosis of a CVLA infection should therefore be made by direct demonstration of the virus in sections of intestinal mucosa or in the feces of scouring pigs.

METHODS AND RESULTS

The immunofluorescent staining technique (IF) on cryostat sections of small intestine from piglets with diarrhea, is routinely used for the

diagnosis of TGE (Pensaert et al., 1968). This technique was adapted for
the diagnosis of CVLA enteritis in young pigs. A hyperimmune serum against
CVLA was raised in a SPF pig and the globulin fraction of the serum was
conjugated with FITC. The specificity of the conjugate was assured by an
inhibition test and by the absence of fluorescence when used on TGEV and
rotaviral containing intestinal sections. The method of the IF technique
is described in the manual. The sensitivity and reliability of the IF as
a diagnostic test in CVLA diarrhea were controlled by staining intestinal
sections of experimentally infected pigs. Thirteen pigs were inoculated
when 2 days old and they were killed at different intervals during the
first 4 days of diarrhea. Specific fluorescence was observed in epithelial
cells covering the small intestinal villi of all the pigs. Intestinal
sections from the jejunum of an uninoculated control pig showed no fluorescence.

We also looked for another diagnostic test for which it was not necessary
to kill the animals. The only test that is working up to now is the electron microscopic examination of the feces of scouring piglets. However,
the detection of a coronavirus particle in the feces of a pig with diarrhea
does not tell us whether it is CVLA or TGE virus. Both particles cannot be
distinguished morphologically. This implies that the EM is only of limited
value for a diagnosis of coronaviral diarrhea in *naturally* infected pigs,
unless it is followed by a specific identification test. Nevertheless,
EM may be very useful in the detection of CVLA in feces of *experimentally*
inoculated piglets. The sensitivity of the EM was tested in piglets experimentally inoculated with CVLA when younger than 20 days by examination
of feces collected at different moments after the onset of diarrhea. The
results are shown in table 1. The highest percentage of positive fecal
samples (maximally 73 %) was obtained at the first day after the beginning
of the diarrhea. Consecutive samples collected from the same pig were
sometimes alternately positive and negative. If several fecal samples from
a same piglet were examined, then the sensitivity of the EM increased to
about 90 %. In another experiment, CVLA particles were never detected in
feces collected from fattening swine having diarrhea after an experimental
inoculation with the CVLA.

CONCLUSIONS

At present, the field diagnosis of a CVLA enteritis can only be made
by the IF technique on cryostat sections of young pigs having diarrhea

for less than 3 days. The sensitivity and the reliability of this technique are very high provided that it is carried out on intestinal segments collected from killed pigs, as described in the manual. The electron microscopic examination of feces is limited in sensitivity and is not specific. It can, therefore, only be used in experimentally inoculated pigs from which several fecal samples should be collected. Fecal samples of naturally infected piglets should be examined by immune EM. The feasability of the immune EM on random collected fecal specimens remains, however, to be established.

We are yet unable to perform the diagnosis of a CVLA infection in pigs older than 2 weeks, until other techniques i.e. serology are established.

TABLE 1 - ELECTRON MICROSCOPICAL EXAMINATION OF FECES FROM 38 PIGLETS, EXPERIMENTALLY INOCULATED WITH THE CORONAVIRUS-LIKE AGENT (CVLA)

Days after onset of diarrhea	Number examined	Number positive for CVLA	(%)
0	37	26	(70)
1	15	11	(73)
2	14	9	(64)
3	13	5	(38)
4	8	0	
5	2	1	

REFERENCES

Pensaert, M.B., Haelterman, E.O. and Burnstein, T. : Diagnosis of Transmissible Gastroenteritis in pigs by means of immunofluorescence. Can. J. Comp. Med. 32 : 555-561, 1968.
Pensaert, M.B. and Debouck, P. : A new coronavirus-like particle associated with diarrhea in swine. Arch. Virol. 58 : 243-247, 1978.
Debouck, P. and Pensaert, M. : Experimental infection of pigs with a new porcine enteric coronavirus, CV 777. Am. J. Vet. Res. 41 : 219-223, 1980.

COMPARISON OF DIAGNOSTIC TECHNIQUES FOR RESEARCH IN NEONATAL DIARRHEA

C. A. Mebus

Plum Island Animal Disease Center, Greenport, New York, 11944 USA

The key word in the assigned topic is "research". This topic can then be broken down into two subdivisions; (1) comparison of currently available diagnostic techniques to recognize outbreaks of diarrhea due to known agents, e.g. rotavirus, coronavirus, E. coli, salmonella, etc. and (2) those techniques which can be used to investigate outbreaks of diarrhea for which an etiologic diagnosis cannot be made using procedures in #1.

Some of the tests described for detection of rotavirus are: direct electron microscopy (EM), immune electron microscopy, fluorescent antibody technique (FAT) on fecal smears and/or sections, immunodiffusion, complement fixation test, fluorescent virus precipitin test, immunoelectroosmophoresis (IEOP), enzyme linked immunosorbent assay (ELISA), radioimmunoassay (RIA), immunofluorescent cell assay, electrophoretic patterns on RNA, solid phase aggregation of coated erythrocytes, and thin layer immunoassay.

The main reason for development of these many tests was a desire to have a reliable and sensitive technique which could be used to screen a large number of specimens quickly, with a minimum of effort, and be available to as many laboratories as possible.

In regards to research, the availability of various diagnostic tests now enables us to compare the sensitivity of those procedures not designed to recognize a specific agent, specifically electron microscopic examination of feces, with those tests based on specific, e.g. immunologic, characteristics, of an agent. Demonstration that a non-specific test can detect a high percentage of infected animals will give confidence to the procedure.

Both direct electron microscopy and immune electron microscopy were two of the first tests used for the diagnosis of enteric viral infections and have been the most frequently used tests to evaluate newly developed procedures. Surprisingly the newer tests were not substantially more sensitive than electron microscopy. Some comparisons of these tests will be reviewed to substantiate this observation.

Peterson, et al., (1976) for rotavirus detection compared the fluorescent virus precipitin test to the immunofluorescent cell test and immune electron microscopic examination on 34 calf and 5 human fecal samples. The results obtained are shown in Table 1.

Spence et al., (1977) compared the counterimmunoelectrophoretic (CIEOP) test to electron microscopic examination for rotavirus on 273 human fecal samples. The assumption was made that EM gave the correct number of positive samples. The CIEOP test detected 86 of 90 EM positive samples and there was one false positive in 183 negative samples.

These results gave the CIEOP test a sensitivity of 95.5% and a specificity of 99.3%. Tufvesson and Johnsson (1976) in 2 similar studies had a 94% and a 100% agreement between EM and CIEOP examination of fecal samples.

Espejo et al., (1977) for the diagnosis of human Rotavirus infection compared the electrophoretic patterns of RNA in partially purified stool virus to electron microscopy. Of 71 fecal samples, 36 were positive by EM and 30 of the 36 were positive by electrophoresis.

Marsolais etal., (1977) compared the fluorescent antibody technique on fecal smears and frozen intestinal sections to electron microscopy on 134 bovine samples for the diagnosis of bovine Rotavirus and calf diarrhea coronavirus infection. These results are shown in Table 2.

Payment et al., (1979) compared immune electron microscopy to the ELISA test for rotavirus on 125 bovine fecal samples. They found that both techniques were equally effective in detecting Rotavirus.

Rhodes et al., (1977) compared on immunodiffusion test to EM and the FAT on fecal smears for detection of rotavirus in 79 calf diarrheic fecal samples. 59% were positive by the immunodiffusion test, 48% were positive by EM, and 20% were positive by FAT (an additional 9% were FAT suspect positive).

Sarkkinen et al., (1979) for Rotavirus detection compared routine electron microscopy, research electron microscopy, and radioimmunoassay on 147 human unconcentrated fecal samples. Research electron microscopy was reexamination of new grids by a more experienced person using higher magnification and spending more time examining each grid. By routine electron microscopy there were 84 positive specimens. By research electron microscopy there were 89 positive specimens, however there was a total of 17 false positive and negative results in the routine electron microscopy findings. Radioimmunoassay detected all of the 89 samples positive by EM and the 6 positive samples in 58 EM negative samples.

Bradburne et al., (1979) for Rotavirus detection compared a solid-phase aggregation of coated erythrocytes to the immuno-flourescent cell culture technique and immune electron microscopy. There was good agreement between all 3 tests.

Wandeler et al., (1980) for Rotavirus detection compared the flourescent antibody technique on fecal smears to the ELISA test using 416 calf fecal samples. 307 samples were negative by both tests; 72 samples were positive by both tests; 3 samples were FAT positive and ELISA negative; and 34 samples were FAT negative and ELISA positive. In addition to the comparative data, there was an interesting observation that rotavirus was almost always associated with diarrhea, and that the ELISA-antigen titer would drop suddenly even though the animal continued to have diarrhea.

Yolken et al., (1977) compared the ELISA test to RIA and EM for detection of Rotavirus in 143 stool samples from children with enteritis and 75 samples from children with other diseases. ELISA detected all 60 specimens positive for Rotavirus by EM and RIA. In another comparision of ELISA, RIA and EM they used serial dilutions of 2% fecal filtrate from a calf experimentally infected with human Rotavirus. EM was negative at a 1:1000 dilution of filtrate. RIA and ELISA were positive at 1:1000, 1:10,000 and negative at 1:100,000.

Simhon et al., (1979) compared the ELISA test to EM for detection of Rotavirus in 247 fecal samples from children with diarrhea. The ELISA test was more sensitive than EM; 5.7 percent of the cases in which there was no visible viral particle were positive by ELISA.

Ellens and DeLeeuw (1977) compared the enzyme-linked immunosorbent assay with electron microscopic and immunoelectro-osmophoretic examination for rotavirus on 98 calf fecal samples and obtained the following results: of the 98 samples, 39 were positive by EM, 30 were positive by IEOP and 49 were positive by ELISA. Of the 39 EM positive cases, 29 were positive by IEOP and 37 by ELISA. They then compared the ELISA test with the IEOP technique on 367 calf fecal samples. 110 samples were positive by the ELISA test; 54 of the 110

positive samples were positive by the IEOP technique and 5 ELISA negative samples were IEOP positive. The very interesting part of this
work was their semi-quantitative EM determinations and dilution
studies to determine sensitivity of the ELISA test. They determined
that the ELISA test was positive when fecal extract contained about
10^5 particles per ml. Purified fecal extract preparation had to
contain about 10^7 particles per ml for a positive ELISA test.
Stated in another way, the ELISA detection limit was about 1 ng of
viral protein per ml. Using fecal homogenates, the ELISA test was
thus about 100 times more sensitive than the IEOP test. These findings
are significant particularly when one realizes that 10^5 particles
per ml is adequate for EM visualization of a virus. This sensitivity
may even be increased to 10^4 particles per ml by using Sharp's
pseudoreplica technique. (Lee, 1980).

In this workshop Scherrer reported comparing EM and ELISA tests
and Grauballe reported comparing EM, IEOP, FAT and ELISA. Both
workers found the ELISA more sensitive than the other tests.

In view of the above comparison of various diagnostic techniques,
large numbers of fecal samples can presently be surveyed by the ELISA
test or radioimmunoassay. One technician using either of these procedures can process over 200 specimens a day and the results are
printed out rather than estimated visually. The disadvantages of the
radioimmunoassay are the cost of equipment and the use of a radioactive isotope. Sophisticated equipment is not required but is
advantageous for performing the ELISA test.

EM examination of feces, for research on diarrhea of unknown
etiology, is the test of choice for several reasons: (1) the procedure is rapid; (2) if the agent happens to be easily inactivated,
it is possible that it may still be observed; (3) a susceptible cell
culture system is not required; (4) no previously prepared biological
reagent is needed, and (5) it is about as sensitive for detecting a
virus as the better immunologic tests. Thus, by using material produced by the patient, electron microscopy may enable detection of an
agent not previously recognized as a cause of diarrhea.

In my opinion, research in neonatal diarrhea is detecting new
etiologic agents of diarrhea. Rapid screening tests are thus useful
for locating herds on which tests for known agents are negative.

A discussion comparing diagnostic techniques for research in neonatal diarrhea in animals would not be complete without mentioning animal inoculation and giving an approach for determining the cause of diarrhea. Once a herd is located, in which the cause of diarrhea cannot be determined, I would take the following approach: (1) collect fecal samples as soon as possible after the onset of diarrhea. The reason for diarrhea is that infection interferes with absorption from the small intestine, therefore there is a high probability that at the onset of diarrhea there should be a large quantity of the etiologic in the feces. (2) Perform direct electron microscopic examination of feces to determine the type(s) of virus(es) present and routine bacteriologic culturing. (3) Attempt to reproduce the disease with whole feces and bacterial free-fecal filtrates. Animal inoculation should be done even if no or few viral particles are observed by electron microscopy. For research in calf diarrhea, all inoculations for initial passages are done in newborn calves by duodenal inoculation. Since diarrhea results from malabsorption of partially digested milk and digestive fluids, it is important that the animals be adequately fed after inoculation. (4) Once diarrhea can be consistently produced in experimental animals, then begins the difficult task of determining the etiologic agent, developing reagents, and isolating the agent in vitro.

SUMMARY

Many diagnostic techniques for rotavirus have been developed with the objective of having a reliable, sensitive, and rapid technique. Published comparisons of these techniques are reviewed in this paper. At present, the ELISA test appears to be the method of choice for examining large number of fecal samples for rotavirus. For research on diarrheal disease, electron microscopic examination of feces is the preferred test. The significance of agents observed in feces, however, must be determined by inoculation of experimental animals.

Table 1 - COMPARISON OF THE FLUORESCENT VIRUS PRECIPITIN TEST WITH
IMMUNOFLUORESCENT CELL TEST AND IMMUNE ELECTRONMICROSCOPY

Fluorescent Virus Precipitin Test	39	14	41
Immunoelectronmicroscopy	39	14	41
Immunofluorescent Cell Test	39	4	12

Table 2 - EXAMINATION OF 134 BOVINE FECAL SAMPLES BY FA AND EM
FOR ROTAVIRUS AND CORONAVIRUS

Rotavirus			Coronavirus		
EM	FA	No. of Cases	EM	FA	No. of Cases
+	+	27	+	+	52
+	-	14	+	-	3
-	+	32	+	NE	23
-	-	61	-	-	42
		134			134

* NE - Not Examined

REFERENCES

Anonymous, 1979a. Detectio n of antigens and IgM antibodies for rapid
diagnosis of viral infections: a WHO Memorandum. Bull. WHO, 57:
925-930.

Bradburne, A.F., Almeida, J.D., Gardner, P.S., Moosai, R.B., Nash,
A.A. and Coombs, R.A.A., 1979b. A solid phase system (SPACE) for
the detection and quantitation of rotavirus in feces. J. Gen.
Virol. 44: 615-623.

Ellens, D.J. and deLeeuw, P.W., 1977a. Enzyme-linked immunosorbent
assay for diagnosis of Rotavirus infections in calves. J.
Clin. Microbiol., 6: 530-532.

Espejo, R.T., Calderon, E. and Gonzalez, N., 1977b. Distinct
    Reovirus-like agents associated with acute infantile
    gastroenteritis. J. Clin. Microbiol., 6: 502–506.

Lee, F.K., Macris, M.P. and Nahmias, A.J., 1980a. Electron microscopy
    for diagnosing viral infection. Lab. Management, 18: 35–39.

Marsolais, G., Assof. R., Montpetit, C. and Marois, P., 1977.
    Diagnosis of viral agents associated with neonatal calf diarrhea.
    Can. J. Comp. Med., 42: 168–171.

Payment, P., Marsolias, G., Trudel, M., Fauvel, M., Lamontagne, L.,
    Assaf, R. and Marois, P., 1979c. Use of electron microscopy and
    an enzyme linked immunosorbent assay for the detection of
    Rotavirus in neonatal calf diarrhea. Can. J. Comp. Med., 43:
    328–329.

Peterson, M.W., Spendlove, R.S. and Smart, R.A., 1976. Detection of
    neonatal calf diarrhea virus, infant Reovirus-like diarrhea
    virus, and a Coronavirus using the fluorescent virus
    precipitin test. J. Clin. Microbiol., 3: 376–377.

Rhodes, M.B., Stair, E.L., McCullough, R.A., McGill, L.D. and Mebus,
    C.A., 1979d. Comparison of results using electron microscopy,
    immunodiffusion and fluorescent antibody analysis to detect
    Rotavirus in Diarrheic fecal samples of calves. Can. J. Comp.
    Med., 43: 84–89.

Sarkkinen, H.K., Halonen, P.E. and Arstila, P.P., 1979e. Comparison
    of four-layer radioimmunoassay and electron microscopy for
    detection of human Rotavirus. J. Med. Virol., 4: 255–260.

Simhon, A., Amato, S., Hernandez, F., Yolken, R.H. and Mata, L.,
    1979f. Diagnostico de Rotavirus por microscopia electronica y el
    ensayo immunosorbente enzima conjugada (ELISA). Bol. Sanit.
    Panam. 86: 391–397.

Spence, L., Fauvel, M., Petro, R. and Bloch, S., 1977c. Comparison of
    counterimmunoelectrophoresis and electromicroscopy for laboratory
    diagnosis of human Reovirus-like agent-associated infantile
    gastroenteritis. J. Clin. Microbiol., 5: 248–249.

Tufvesson, B. and Johnsson, T., 1976. Immunoelectroosmophoresis for
    detection of Reo-like virus methodology and comparison with
    electron microscopy. Wandeler, A., Kunzli, C., Kunz, U. and

Steck, F., 1980b. Rotavirus infections in calves. Experientia,
    36:    498. Yolken, R.H., Kim, H.W., Clem, T., Wyatt, R.G.,
    Kalica,A.R., Chanock, R.M. and Kapikian, A.Z. 1977d.
    Enzyme-linked immunosorbent assay (ELISA) gastroenteritis.
Lancet, 2: 263–267. Wandeler, A., Kunzli, C., Kunz, U. and Steck, F.,
    1980. Rotavirus infections in calves. Experientia, 36:
    498.
Yolken, R.H., Kim, H.W., Clem, T., Wyatt, R.G., Kalica, A.R., Chanock,
    R.M. and Kapikian, A.Z. 1977. Enzyme-linked immunosorbent
    assay (ELISA)for detection of human Reovirus-like agent of
    infantile gastroenteritis. Lancet, 2:   263–267.

ELECTRON MICROSCOPY FOR THE DETECTION OF BOVINE AND PORCINE ROTAVIRUSES, BOVINE ENTERIC CORONAVIRUS, CALICIVIRUS-LIKE AGENTS AND ASTROVIRUSES IN FAECES.

Laboratory manual of the Agricultural Research Council's Institute for Research on Animal Diseases, Compton, Nr. Newbury, Berks., UK.

Reference: J.C. Bridger, G.N. Woode and A. Meyling: Isolation of corona-viruses from neonatal calf diarrhoea in Great Britain and Denmark. Vet. Microbiol. 3, 101-113, 1978.

The method is based on differential centrifugation followed if neces-sary by centrifugation through a sucrose cushion.

1. Mix well 5 g of faeces with 15 ml PBSa (pH 7.2).
2. Clarify the faecal suspension by centrifugation at 3,000 to 8,000 g for 30 min and pour off the supernatant fluid.
3. Repeat step 2 if necessary.
4. Centrifuge the supernatant fluid at 100,000 g for 1 h and resuspend the resulting pellet in a few drops of PBSa using a wide needle and syringe to aid resuspension. If the pellets appear to be too large or are grossly contaminated, proceed to step 5..
5. Layer the resuspended high speed pellet on to 4 ml of 40% (w/w) sucrose solution or on to 4 ml 40% sucrose solution plus 5 ml 30% sucrose solu-tion. Centrifuge at 83,000 g for 2 h and resuspend the resulting pellet in 0.2 ml PBSa.
6. Place a drop of the resuspended pellet, or a suitable dilution of it, on a carbon-formvar electron microscope grid, blot off the excess and stain with 2% potassium phototungstate pH 6.0.
7. Grids should be examined for 10-15 min before a negative result can be reported. In this time it should be possible to thoroughly examine at least 5 good squares of a 400 mesh grid.
N.B. For additional information on diagnosis of enteric infections by EM, see McNulty 1980, these proceedings.

DETECTION OF PORCINE AND BOVINE ROTAVIRUSES IN FAECES
BY INFECTIVITY ASSAY IN CELL CULTURE

Laboratory manual of the Agricultural Research Council's Institute for Research on Animal Diseases, Compton, Nr. Newbury, Berks., UK.

REFERENCE
Bridger, J.C. and Brown, J.M.: Development of immunity to porcine rotavirus in piglets protected from disease by bovine colostrum.   To be published.

METHOD
1.   Make 10% suspensions of faeces in Eagle's maintenance medium.
2.   Centrifuge at 8 000 g for 30 min and pour off supernatant fluids.
3.   Filter supernatant fluids through clarifier and 0.45 µm filters (Millipore).
4.   Make serial ten-fold dilutions of filtered suspensions in Eagle's maintenance medium in duplicate.
5.   Inoculate 0.1 ml of each dilution into 4 wells of a micro-titre plate (Sterilin) containing 48-hour-old confluent monolayers of LLC-MK$_2$ cells grown in Eagle's medium with 10% foetal calf serum.
6.   Centrifuge inoculated plates at 300 g for 1 hour and incubate for 18 hours at 37°C.
7.   Shake off medium from cultures, add 80% acetone (diluted in distilled water) at -20°C, leave 10 mins at room temperature.
8.   Shake off acetone, dry plates at 37°C.
9.   Add 1 drop of a suitable dilution in PBSa of antiserum to bovine rotavirus and leave at room temperature for one hour.
10.   Shake off antiserum and wash plates 4 times with PBSa.
11.   Add 1 drop of a suitable dilution of rabbit anti-bovine immuno-globulin-FITC conjugate (Nordic) and leave at room temperature for one hour.
12.   Shake off FITC-conjugate, wash 4 times with PBSa and read inverted plates using an incident-light fluorescence microscope.   Record each well for the presence of individual fluorescent cells.

13. Determine end-points using the Reed & Muench equation: up to 10^8 TCD_{50} per gram of faeces can be detected.

INGREDIENTS

1) Eagle's maintenance medium: Eagle's minimal essential medium containing 0.1% sodium bicarbonate, 100 units benzyl penicillin, 100 µg streptomycin sulphate and 25 µg mycostatin per ml of culture fluid.

2) Antiserum to bovine rotavirus: The serum was produced in a 7-day-old gnotobiotic calf inoculated with a bovine rotavirus obtained from an outbreak of diarrhoea and passaged serially 7 times in gnotobiotic calves. The calf developed diarrhoea and 23 days after the oral inoculation received an intravenous inoculation of a faecal filtrate containing bovine rotavirus; four days later the calf was bled out. The antiserum obtained had a neutralisation titre of 1:1 280 to the cell culture-adapted Compton, UK, isolate of bovine rotavirus (Bridger and Woode, Br. Vet. J. 131: 528-535, 1975).

NOTE: Additional modifications may increase the sensitivity of the test - see the presentation 'Cell culture techniques for the identification of enteric viruses - present possibilities' - J.C. Bridger.

DETECTION OF BOVINE ASTROVIRUSES IN FAECES
BY INFECTIVITY ASSAY IN CELL CULTURE

Laboratory manual of the Agricultural Research Council's Institute for Research on Animal Diseases, Compton, Nr. Newbury, Berks., UK.

REFERENCE
Ormerod, E. and Bridger, J.C. (unpublished).

METHOD
1. Make 10% suspensions of faeces in PBSa, pH 7.2.
2. Allow to stand for 30 min and pipette off the supernatant fluid.
3. Inoculate 0.1 ml of the supernatant fluid on to confluent primary calf kidney cultures grown in microtitre trays (Sterilin) and incubate for one hour at 37°C.
4. Remove the inoculum and wash cells with PBSa.
5. Add 0.1 ml Eagle's maintenance medium and incubate for 18 hours at 37°C.
6. Fix and stain as described for 'Detection of porcine and bovine rotaviruses in faeces by infectivity assay in cell culture', points 7 to 13, but using convalescent antiserum to bovine astrovirus produced in a gnotobiotic calf. Up to 10^7 $TCID_{50}$ per gram of faeces can be obtained from field material. Toxicity to cells can be avoided by diluting the inoculum.

INGREDIENTS
Eagle's maintenance medium: Eagle's minimal essential medium containing 0.1% sodium bicarbonate, 5% foetal calf serum, 200 µg/ml benzyl penicillin, streptomycin sulphate and kanamycin.

DETECTION OF BOVINE ENTERIC CORONAVIRUSES IN FAECES
BY INOCULATION OF TRACHEAL ORGAN CULTURES

Laboratory manual of the Agricultural Research Council's Institute for
Research on Animal Diseases, Compton, Nr. Newbury, Berks., UK.

REFERENCES

Stott, E.J., Thomas, L.H., Bridger, J.C. and Jebbett, N.J.: Replication
     of a bovine coronavirus in organ cultures of foetal trachea.
     Vet. Microbiol. 1: 65-69, 1976.
Bridger, J.C., Woode, G.N. and Meyling, A.: Isolation of coronaviruses
     from neonatal calf diarrhoea in Great Britain and Denmark.
     Vet. Microbiol. 3: 101-113, 1978.

METHOD

1. Prepare tracheal rings from bovine foetuses between 5 and 6 months
   of gestation.   Depending on size, put 1 ring per tube with 1 ml
   Eagle's maintenance medium or up to 5 rings per bottle with 5 ml of
   medium.

2. To infect, immerse rings in a mixture of equal volumes of an 0.45 μ
   faecal filtrate and 0.5 ml of Eagle's maintenance medium for 1.5
   hours at 37°C.

3. Remove unadsorbed virus by washing the rings with 5 ml medium,
   add a suitable volume of maintenance medium and roll at 37°C.

4. Change the medium every 3 or 4 days for up to 21 days and assay for
   haemagglutinating activity.

5. Remove one ring 10 and 21 days after inoculation and stain for
   immunofluorescent antigens.

HAEMAGGLUTINATION TEST

1. Add 1% (v/v) washed rat erythrocytes to samples diluted in
   microtitre plates with PBSa containing 0.1% bovine serum albumin.

2. Read end-points after the erythrocytes have been allowed to settle
   for 1-1.5 hours at 4°C.

IMMUNOFLUORESCENCE OF TRACHEAL RINGS

1. Freeze tracheal rings in liquid nitrogen and section in a cryostat.

2.   Fix in acetone for 10 minutes.

3.   Stain by the direct method with fluorescein-conjugated rabbit
     antiserum to the American bovine enteric coronavirus or by the
     indirect method with convalescent antisera and fluorescein-
     conjugated rabbit anti-bovine gamma globulin antiserum.

4.   Examine for immunofluorescent antigens.

INGREDIENTS

Eagle's maintenance medium: Eagle's minimal essential medium containing
0.14% sodium bicarbonate, 0.09% bovine plasma albumin, 5% tryptose
phosphate broth, 100 units/ml penicillin, 100 μg/ml streptomycin,
250 μg/ml ampicillin, 100 μg/ml kanamycin, 25 μg/ml mycostatin, and
30mM HEPES buffer adjusted to pH 7.2 with 1N NaOH.

ROTAVIRUS NEUTRALISATION TEST IN CELL CULTURE
BY A FLUORESCENT FOCUS REDUCTION TEST

Laboratory manual of the Agricultural Research Council's Institute for
Research on Animal Diseases, Compton, Nr. Newbury, Berks., UK.

REFERENCE

Adapted from: Thouless, M.E., Bryden, A.S., Flewett, T.H., Woode, G.N.,
Bridger, J.C., Snodgrass, D.R. and Herring, J.A.: Serological
relationships between rotaviruses from different species as studied
by complement fixation and neutralisation. Arch. Virol. 53:
287-294, 1977.

The method is based on the observation that wild-type rotaviruses will
infect cell cultures to produce single-cell immunofluorescence and that
the infectivity can be neutralised by rotavirus antiserum.

METHOD

1. Make a ten-fold dilution of the serum to be assayed in Eagle's
    maintenance medium and heat at $56^{\circ}C$ for 30 min.

2. Make doubling dilutions (50 µl in 50 µl of Eagle's medium) in
    duplicate from the heat-inactivated 1:10 serum dilutions.

3. Add 50 µl of a rotavirus suspension (diluted in Eagle's medium to
    contain 100-200 fluorescent foci per 5 µl) to each doubling dilution
    and incubate for 2 hours at $37^{\circ}C$.

4. Add 10 µl of the virus-serum mixtures to 48-hour-old confluent
    LLC-MK$_2$ monolayers grown in microtitre trays and maintained with
    0.1 ml Eagle's maintenance medium: inoculate 3 wells per antiserum
    dilution.

5. Centrifuge, incubate and stain inoculated plates as described for
    'Detection of bovine and porcine rotaviruses in faeces by
    infectivity assay in cell culture' points 6 to 12.

6. Count the number of fluorescent cells per well and determine the
    antiserum dilution which gives a 50% reduction in the number of
    fluorescent cells.

INGREDIENTS

Eagle's maintenance medium: Eagle's minimal essential medium containing
0.1% sodium bicarbonate, 100 units of benzyl penicillin, 100 µg
streptomycin sulphate and 25 µg mycostatin per ml of culture fluid.

MANUAL I

ELISA FOR THE DETECTION AND QUANTITATION OF ROTAVIRUS IN FAECES

R. Scherrer[*], Chantal Feynerol[*] and R. L'Haridon[**]

[*] Station de Recherches de Virologie et d'Immunologie INRA
78 850 - Thiverval-Grignon, France
[**]Present address : Laboratoire de Pathologie du Bétail ENV
94 701 - Maisons-Alfort, France.

(Modification of the technique described by R. Scherrer and S.Bernard 1977)

PRINCIPLE OF THE ASSAY

The wells in a polystyrene plate (solid phase) are coated with a specific anti rotavirus Ig preparation (sensitization of the wells). Plates are then washed in order to remove immunoglobulins that are not adsorbed. Upon addition of faecal extracts, rotavirus particles and/or antigens, if they are present, will be trapped by the immobilized antibodies. After removal of unbound material, (washing) a conjugate consisting of antirotavirus antibodies coupled to alkalin phosphatase, is added in the wells ; this conjugate will react with any rotaviral antigen already trapped in the wells. A further washing removes excess conjugate and finally, the bound conjugate is visualized by adding the enzyme substrate (p-nitrophenylphosphate).

1. Preparation of faecal extracts

- Homogenize one volume of faeces in four volumes of PBS pH 7.4 (1)
- Clarify by centrifugation at 2500 g for 20 min.
- Collect the supernatant and dilute an aliquot with one volume of
  PBS-Tween-Sodium azide (3) (dilution of faeces 1:10)

2. Preparation of rabbit (or goat) anti rotavirus Ig.

- The rabbit anti rotavirus Ig preparation used in the test was obtained from a gnotobiotic rabbit inoculated intramuscularly with purified bovine rotavirus (mixture of double-shelled and single-shelled particles) (J. Cohen 1977) in complete Freund's adjuvant. The rabbit was reinoculated intraveneously 4 weeks later with purified virus alone. Anti rotavirus activity of the serum was checked every two days by indirect immunofluorescence test on preinfected calf-kidney cell-cultures (Thiverval bovine-

rotavirus strain)(R. L'Haridon and R. Scherrer 1976) and the rabbit bled
6 to 8 days after the second injection. (IIF titre : 20,000).

The immunoglobulins in one volume of serum were precipitated twice
with Na_2SO_4 (36 % and 34 %), redissolved in one volume of PBS and dialysed
against PBS. Storage is at - 80°C in small aliquots.

The goat anti rotavirus Ig preparation was obtained in the same way
from a seronegative 8 months-old goat. The anti rotavirus titre of the
serum was 35,000 by IIF test.

The optimal concentrations of rabbit or goat anti rotavirus Ig preparations, for coating the plates, were determined by checkerboard titra-
tions.

3. Preparation of anti rotavirus conjugate.

The conjugate was prepared by coupling rabbit anti rotavirus Ig with
alkaline phosphatase (8) using glutaraldehyde, according to the technique
described by E. Engvall and P. Perlmann, 1972. The conjugate, diluted
1:100, is stored in 50 mM Tris buffer pH 8.0 containing $MgCl_2.6H_2O$ (1 mM),
NaN_3 (3 mM) and HSA (3g % w/v).

The optimal dilution of the conjugate in the assay is 1:37,000 as
determined by checkerboard titration.

PERFORMANCE OF THE ASSAY

1. Preparation of microplates.

(Disposable polystyrene plates - Ref. Linbro-1S-FB-96 ; Flow laboratories)
- Pretreat the wells with a 1 % glutaraldehyde solution in distilled
  water (100 µl per well) and incubate for 1 hour at 4°C.
- Wash thoroughly with distilled water, six times.

(This step is not absolutely necessary, however it was shown that pretreatment with glutaraldehyde is beneficial, probably by modifying the adsorption capacity of the plastic).

2. Coating the plates with anti rotavirus Ig preparation.

(Sensitization of the plates)
- Dilute appropriately the anti rotavirus Ig preparation in carbonate-
  bicarbonate buffer pH 9.6 (4)
  (Standard rabbit Ig 1:2,000 or standard goat Ig 1 : 7,000)
- Add 100 µl per well and cover the plate with plate sealing tape
  (Titertek)
- Incubate for 17 hours at 20°C
- Wash with PBS-Tween (2) three times

Washing procedure : The content of the wells are thrown out, the wells filled up with PBS-Tween using a squeeze bottle and the plate left for two minutes. The washing solution is then thrown out and the plate tapped, upside down against soft absorbent paper. This washing procedure is repeated twice more.

(At this stage, the coated plates may be stored at 4°C during six to eight weeks, without loss of anti rotavirus activity. For this purpose, wash the plates with distilled water, allow them to air-dry and store them at 4°C, avoiding humidity).

3. Incubation with faecal samples and standard controls.

- Prepare the dilutions of the faecal extracts (1:10, 1:100, 1:1000, 1:10 000), of the positive reference (6) (1:10, 1:100, 1:1000) and of the negative control (7) (1:10) using PBS-Tween-Sodium azide.
- Fill the wells with 100 μl volumes as follows :

  Row 1 : using PBS-Tween-Sodium azide (for blanking)

  Row 2 : using the positive reference and the negative control
  (each dilution in duplicate)

  Row 3 to 12 : using 10 faecal samples (each dilution in duplicate)
- Cover the plate and incubate 2 hours at 20°C
- Wash with PBS-Tween, three times.

4. Incubation with anti rotavirus conjugate.

- Prepare the dilution of conjugate (1 : 37,000 in PBS-Tween)
- Add 100 µl per well and cover the plate
- Incubate for 2,5 hours at 20°C
- Wash with PBS-Tween, four times

5. Incubation with substrate solution.

- Prepare the substrate solution (p-nitrophenylphosphate 1 mg per ml in diethanolamine buffer pH 9.8 (5)
- Add 100 μl per well and cover the plate
- Incubate for 60 min. at 37°C.
- Stop the reaction by adding 50 µl 3M NaOH in each well.
- Read the test in the Titertek[R] Multiskan (A 405).

6. Interpretation

. Faecal samples are considered positif for rotavirus if the A 405 value (mean of two test wells) is $\geqslant 0.2$ (P / N ratio $\geqslant 5$)

. For quantitation, express the relative titre of a sample as the reciprocal of the dilution corresponding to A 405 of 0.2.

BUFFERS AND REAGENTS

(1) PHOSPHATE BUFFERED SALINE (PBS) pH 7.4

NaCl	8.0 g
KH_2PO_4	0.2 g
$Na_2HPO_4 \cdot 12\ H_2O$	2.9 g
KCl	0.2 g
H_2O	A.D. 1000 ml

(2) PBS TWEEN

$Tween_{20}$	0.5 ml
PBS pH 7.4	A.D. 1000 ml

(3) PBS-TWEEN-SODIUM AZIDE

$Tween_{20}$	0.5 ml
NaN_3	0.2 g
PBS pH 7.4	A.D. 1000 ml

(4) CARBONATE-BICARBONATE BUFFER pH 9.6

Na_2CO_3	1.59 g	(15 mM)
$NaHCO_3$	2.93 g	(35 mM)
NaN_3	0,2 g	(3 mM)
H_2O	A.D. 1000 ml	

(5) DIETHANOLAMINE BUFFER pH 9.8

Diethanolamine $HN(CH_2CH_2OH)_2$ (Fluka, code 31590) 97 ml; $MgCl_2 6H_2O$, 0.1 g Add about 800 ml distilled water and adjust the pH to 9.8 with 1 M HCl ; than add distilled water up to 1000 ml. Store at 4°C in the dark.

(6) POSITIVE REFERENCE

Mixture of purified single-shelled and double-shelled rotavirus particles (200 μg virus in PBS-Tween)

(7) NEGATIVE CONTROL

Faecal specimen from a calf not containing rotavirus as tested by electron microscopy and ELISA.

(8) ALKALINE PHOSPHATASE

Type VII ; 1140 units/mg protein (Sigma, code P-4502)

REFERENCES

Cohen, J. : Ribonucleic acid polymerase activity associated with puri-
    fied calf rotavirus. J. Gen. Virol. 36 : 395-402, 1977.
Engvall, E. and Perlmann, P. : Enzyme-linked immunosorbent assay, ELISA.
    III. Quantitation of specific antibodies by enzyme-labeled anti
    immunoglobulin in antigen coated tubes. J. Immunol. 109 : 129-135,
    1972.
L'Hàridon, R. and Scherrer, R. : Culture in vitro du rotavirus associé
    aux diarrhées néonatales du veau. Ann. Rech. Vét. 7 (4) : 373-381,
    1976.
Scherrer, R. and Bernard, S. : Application d'une technique immunoenzymo-
    logique (ELISA) à la détection du rotavirus bovin et des anticorps
    dirigés contre lui. Ann. Microbiol. (Institut Pasteur) 128 A : 499-
    510, 1977.

MANUAL II

ELISA FOR THE DETECTION AND TITRATION

OF BOVINE ANTI ROTAVIRUS Ig IN SERA

R. L'Haridon[*], R. Scherrer[**] and C. Feynerol[**]

[*] Present address : Laboratoire de Pathologie du Bétail ENV

94 701 - Maisons-Alfort , France

[**]Station de Recherches de Virologie et d'Immunologie INRA

78 850 - Thiverval-Grignon, France.

PRINCIPLE OF THE ASSAY

The wells in a polystyrene plate are coated with purified rotavirus particles (sensitization of the wells). Plates are washed to remove virus not adsorbed. Upon addition of a bovine serum sample, anti rotavirus antibodies, if present, will be trapped by the rotaviral antigens. After removal of unbound components, a conjugate consisting of anti bovine-IgG (H and L) antibodies coupled to alkaline phosphatase, is added in the wells. This conjugate will react with anti rotaviral bovine-Ig already trapped on the wells. A further washing removes excess conjugate, and finally the bound conjugate is visualized by adding the enzyme substrate (p-Nitrophenylphosphate).

SPECIFIC REAGENTS

- Anti-bovine IgG conjugate.

Goat anti bovine-IgG (heavy and light chains) was obtained from Miles Laboratories (Code 61-079). The product was coupled to alkaline phosphatase (8), using glutaraldehyde, according to the technique of E. Engvall and P. Perlmann 1972. The conjugate is stored at 4°C in the dark (dilution 1:100 in 50 mM Tris buffer pH 8.0 containing $MgCl_2.6H_2O$ (1 mM), NaN_3 (3 mM) and HSA (3 g % w/v).

Before and after coupling with alkaline phosphatase, the preparation has been tested for absence of anti rotavirus activity, by indirect immunofluorescence test as described by R. L'Haridon and R. Scherrer 1976, using an anti goat immunofluorescent serum, and by ELISA.

- Standard controls.

. Positive reference serum

Obtained from a seropositive cow (Neutralization titre : 15,000)

(see manual V for neutralization test)

Negative reference serum

Obtained from a colostrum deprived calf.

PERFORMANCE OF THE ASSAY

1. Preparation of microplates

(Pretreatment and sensitization)

- Pretreat the wells with glutaraldehyde and wash (same technique as in manual I)
- Add 100 µl per well of a purified rotavirus suspension (J. Cohen 1977) adjusted to 5 µg virus per ml. (double-shelled particles ; single-shelled particles or mixtures of both may be used) in Pipes buffer pH 6.3 (9).
- Cover the plate with plate sealing tape.
- Incubate for 6 hours at 37°C.
- Wash with PBS-Tween (2), three times.

2. Incubation with test samples and standard controls.

- Prepare two fold serial dilutions of the test samples using PBS-Tween-Sodium azide (3), starting at the dilution 1:20
- Dilute the positive reference serum and the negative reference serum in the same way
- Add 100 µl of each dilution per well (in duplicate)
- Cover the plate and incubate 17 hours at 37°C
- Wash with PBS-Tween, three times.

3. Incubation with anti bovine-IgG conjugate.

- Prepare the dilution of conjugate using PBS-Tween (the optimal dilution of the conjugate in the assay is 1 : 2700 as determined by checkerboard titration)
- Add 100 µl per well and cover the plate
- Incubate for 2.5 hours at 37°C
- Wash with PBS-Tween, four times.

4. Incubation with substrate solution and reading.

(same technique as in manual I)

- Express the titre as the reciprocal of the serum dilution corresponding to an A 405 of 0.2

BUFFERS AND CHEMICALS

(2), (3) and (8) see Manual I

(9) PIPES BUFFER 0.05M pH 6.3

Pipes (piperazine-N$_1$N'-bis (2 ethane sulfonic acid)   15.12 g

NaCl   8.0 g

Dissolve in about 500 ml distilled water adjusted to pH 8.0 with 10 N NaOH. Then adjust the pH to 6.3 with HCl. Add distilled water up to 1000 ml.

REFERENCES

Cohen, J. : Ribonucleic acid polymerase activity associated with puri-fied calf rotavirus. J. Gen. Virol. 36 : 395-402, 1977.

Engvall, E. and Perlmann, P. : Enzyme-linked immunosorbent assay, ELISA. III – Quantitation of specific antibodies by enzyme-labeled anti immunoglobulin in antigen-coated tubes. J. Immunol. 109 : 129-135, 1972.

L'Haridon, R. and Scherrer, R. : Culture in vitro du rotavirus associé aux diarrhées néonatales du veau. Ann. Rech. Vét. 7 (4) : 373-381, 1976.

MANUAL III

ELISA FOR THE DETECTION OF PIG ANTI ROTAVIRUS

IgG, IgA AND IGM IN FAECES

G. Corthier[*], J. Franz[**] and R. Scherrer[***]

[*] Laboratoire de Pathologie Porcine INRA,
78850 Thiverval-Grignon, France.

[**] Institut de Recherches vétérinaires, Brno,
Tchécoslovaquie.

[***] Station de Virologie et d'Immunologie, INRA,
78850 Thiverval-Grignon, France.

PRINCIPLE OF THE ASSAY

The wells in a polystyrene plate are coated with purified rotavirus particles (sensitization of the wells). Plates are washed to remove virus not adsorbed. Upon addition of a faecal extract, antirotavirus antibodies of the IgG, IgA or IgM class (if present) will be trapped by the rotaviral antigens. After removal of unbound material, class-specific anti porcine-Ig (H chains) antibodies (either anti IgG, or anti IgA or anti IgM antibodies, rised in rabbits) are added to the wells. A further washing removes unbound antibodies. The bound antibodies are then detected using a conjugate consisting of antibodies directed against rabbit immunoglobulins and coupled to alkaline phosphatase. After washing, the bound conjugate is visualized by adding the enzyme substrate (p-Nitrophenylphosphate).

SPECIFIC REAGENTS

- Rabbit anti porcine IgG, IgA or IgM

The different antisera were prepared in rabbits hyperimmunized with pure porcine IgG or IgA or IgM (H chains) preparations (J.F. Bourne (1969); J. Curtis and J.F. Bourne (1971)). The anti IgG and anti IgA sera were absorbed to IgM coupled to sepharose 4B (for isolation of anti IgG and anti IgA H-chains antibodies) and the anti IgM serum to IgG and α_2 macroglobuline, coupled to sepharose 4B (for isolation of anti IgM H-chains antibodies). The class specificity of the different preparations was assessed by non competitive ELISA, using alternatively pure IgG, pure IgA and pure IgM from naturally rotavirus infected pigs. (G. Corthier and J. Franz ; in preparation).

- Anti rabbit-Ig conjugate

The antibodies were prepared in a pig, hyperimmunized with purified rabbit IgG (N. Harboe and A. Ingild, 1973). The serum was absorbed to insolubilized rabbit immunoglobulins, eluted with 0.1 M glycine-HCl buffer pH 2.8 and finally dialysed against PBS.

Coupling of the antibodies with alkaline phosphatase was performed according to the technique described by S. Avrameas (1969).

- Standard controls

Detection and quantitation of anti rotavirus IgG

Positif control : pure IgG having anti rotavirus activity, obtained from naturally infected pigs.

Negative controls :

   a) pure IgM and IgA having anti rotavirus activity

   b) faecal extract obtained from SPF pigs not containing anti rotavirus IgG, IgA and IgM.

Detection and quantitation of anti rotavirus IgA

Positif control : pure IgA having anti rotavirus activity

Negative controls :

   a) pure IgG and IgM having anti rotavirus activity

   b) same as above

Detection and quantitation of anti rotavirus IgM

Positif control : pure IgM having anti rotavirus activity

Negative control :

   a) pure IgA and IgG having anti rotavirus activity

   b) same as above.

PERFORMANCE OF THE ASSAY

1. Preparation of the microplates

   (Pretreatment and sensitization)

     - Pretreat the wells with glutaraldehyde and wash
       (same technique as in manual I)

     - Add 100 μl per well of a purified rotavirus suspension
       (J. Cohen, 1977) containing single-shelled particles adjusted to
       a concentration of 2 μg/ml in carbonate-bicarbonate buffer PH 9.6
       (4).

     - Cover the plate and incubate for 3 hours at 37°C

     - Wash with PBS-Tween (2), three times.

2. Incubation with test samples and standard controls

- Prepare three fold serial dilutions of the test samples in
  PBS-Tween-Sodium azide (3) starting at the dilution 1 : 10
  (for preparation of faecal extracts, see manual I)
- Prepare in the same way the positive and the negative controls.
- Fill the wells with 100 µl volumes of each dilution (in duplicate)
- Cover the plates and incubate overnight at 20°C
- Wash with PBS-Tween, three times.

3. Incubation with class-specific anti porcine-Ig preparations

- Adjust the concentration of all preparations to 10 µg immuno-
  globulins/ml (protein concentration estimated by A 280 value)
  using PBS-Tween.
- Add 100 µl per well
- Cover the plate and incubate for three hours at 37°C
- Wash with PBS-Tween, three times

4. Incubation with pig anti rabbit-Ig conjugate

- Fill the wells with 100 µl volumes of the conjugate (optimal
  concentration of the conjugate is 1.2 µg/ml measured as Ig by
  absorbancy at 280 nm)
- Cover the plate and incubate for three hours at 37°C
- Wash with PBS-Tween four times.

5. Incubation with substrate solution and reading

(same technique as in manual I)

Interpretation

. Faecal samples are considered positif for anti rotavirus IgG or
  IgA or IgM if the A 405 value is $\geqslant$ 0.2 (P/N ratio $\geqslant$ 5)
. For quantitation, express the relative titre of a sample as the
  reciprocal of the dilution corresponding to A 405 of 0.2

BUFFERS AND CHEMICALS

(see manual I)

REFERENCES

Avrameas, S. : Coupling of enzymes to proteins with glutaraldehyde. Use of
  conjugates for the detection of antigens and antibodies. Immunoche-
  mistry 6: 43-52, 1969.
Bourne, J.F. : IgA immunoglobulin from porcin milk. Bioch. Biophys. Acta.
  181 : 485-487, 1969.
Cohen, J. : Ribonucleic Acid Polymerase activity associated with purified
  calf rotavirus. J. Gen. Virol. 36 : 395-402, 1977.

Curtis, J. Bourne, J.F. : Immunoglobulin quantitation in sow serum,colostrum and milk. Biochim. Biophys. Acta. 236 : 319-332, 1971.
Harboe, N., Ingild, A. : Immunisation, isolation of immunoglobulins, estimation of antibody titer. Scand. J. Immunol. 2 : 161-164, 1973.

MANUAL IV

ELISA FOR THE DETECTION OF ROTAVIRUS/ANTIBODY COMPLEXES
IN PORCINE FAECES.

G. Corthier [*] and R. Scherrer [**]

[*]Laboratoire de Pathologie porcine, INRA

78850 - Thiverval-Grignon, France.

[**]Station de Virologie et d'Immunologie, INRA

78850 - Thiverval-Grignon, France.

PRINCIPLE OF THE ASSAY

The wells in a polystyrene plate are coated with an anti rotavirus rabbit-IgG preparation (sensitization of the wells). Plates are washed in order to remove IgG that are not adsorbed. Upon addition of a faecal extract, rotavirus particles and/or antigens that are not complexed with antibodies or only underline partially complexed (so that they can still react antigenically) will be trapped (if present) by the rabbit antibodies immobilized on the solid phase. After removal of unbound material, a conjugate consisting of anti pig-Ig (L chains) antibodies, coupled to alkaline phosphatase, is added in the wells. This conjugate will react with any anti rotavirus porcine-immunoglobulin already complexed with virus. A further washing removes excess conjugate and finally the bound conjugate is visualized by adding the enzyme substrate (p-Nitrophenyl-phosphate).

SPECIFIC REAGENTS

- Rabbit anti rotavirus IgG

The antibody preparation was obtained from a rabbit hyperimmunized with purified pig rotavirus (purification according to the technique described by J. Cohen, 1977, for bovine rotavirus) in complete Freund's adjuvant (three intramuscular injections at four weeks interval). The serum, collected 8 days after the third injection was precipitated with ammonium sulfate (50 %) and then IgG were purified by ion exchange on a DEAE Sephadex column (N. Harboe and A. Ingild, 1973).

- Rabbit anti pig-Ig (L chains) preparation

   The antibody preparation was obtained from a rabbit hyperimmunized
   with pure pig IgG (J.F. Bourne, 1969). The antiserum was then
   absorbed with pure IgM, insolubilized with glutaraldehyde (S.
   Avrameas and T. Ternynck 1969). The anti L immunoglobulins were
   then eluted with 0.1 M glycine-HCl buffer pH 2.8 (S. Avrameas 1969)
   and dialysed against PBS.

   Coupling with alkaline phosphatase was performed according to the
   technique described by S. Avrameas, 1969.

- Standard controls

   . Negative control :

      Suspension of purified single-shelled bovine rotavirus particles

   . Positive control :

      Mixture of purified bovine rotavirus particles with antiserum
      against the pig rotavirus OSU strain (E.H. Bohl et al., 1978)

PERFORMANCE OF THE ASSAY

1. Preparation of microplates

   (pretreatment and sensitization)

   - pretreat the wells with glutaraldehyde and wash (same technique
     as in manual I)
   - add 100 μl per well of rabbit anti rotavirus IgG preparation
     (5 μg IgG per ml in carbonate-bicarbonate buffer pH 9.6 (4)
   - cover the plate and incubate for three hours at 37°C
   - wash with PBS-Tween (2), three times.

2. Incubation with faecal extracts and standard controls

   - prepare three fold serial dilutions of the faecal extracts
     using PBS-Tween-Sodium azide (3) (for preparation of faecal
     extracts see manual I)
   - prepare in the same way the positive and the negative controls
   - fill the wells with 100 μl volumes of each dilution (in duplicate)
   - cover the plate and incubate overnight at 20°C
   - wash with PBS Tween, three times.

3. Incubation with anti pig Ig (L chains) conjugate

   - adjust the concentration of the conjugate to 1.2 μg Ig per ml
     (measured as Ig by absorbancy at 280 nm) using PBS-Tween
   - add 100 μl per well
   - cover the plate and incubate for 3 hours at 37°C

- Wash with PBS-Tween, four times.

4. Incubation with substrate solution and reading

(same technique as in manual I)

INTERPRETATION

Faecal samples are considered positif for rotavirus immune complexes if the A 405 value is ≥ 0.2 (P/N ration ≥ 5).

BUFFERS AND REAGENTS

(see Manual I)

REFERENCES

Avrameas, S., Ternynck, T. : The cross linking of protein with glutaral-dehyde and its use for preparation of immunoadsorbents. Immunoche-mistry 6 : 53-66, 1969.

Avrameas, S. : Coupling of enzymes to proteins with glutaraldehyde. Use of conjugates for the detection of antigens and antibodies. Immuno-chemistry 6 : 43-52, 1969

Bohl, E.H., Kohler, E.M., S.aif, L.J., Cross, R.F., Agnes, A.G., Theil, K.W. : Rotavirus as a cause of diarrhea in pigs. J. Am. Vet. Med. Ass. 172 : 458-463, 1978.

Bourne, J.F. : IgA immunoglobulin from porcin milk. Biochim. Biophys. Acta. 181 : 485-487, 1969.

Cohen, J. : Ribonucleic acid polymerase activity associated with purified calf rotavirus. J. Gen. Virol. 36 : 395-402, 1977

Harboe, N., Ingild, A. : Immunisation, isolation of immunoglobulins, es-timation of antibody titer. Scand. J. Immunol. 2 : 161-164, 1973.

MANUAL V

NEUTRALIZING ANTIBODY PLAQUE ASSAY FOR BOVINE ROTAVIRUS

J.F. Vautherot, J. Cohen, Chantal Feynerol and R. Scherrer
Station de Recherches de Virologie et d'Immunologie INRA ,
78 850 - Thiverval-Grignon, France.

PREPARATION OF CELL CULTURES

- Prepare confluent monolayers of MA 104 cells (Foetal Rhesus monkey kidney) in disposable tissue-culture plates (Costar - 6 wells; code 3506; 205 Broadway. Cambridge, Mass.).
  For this purpose seed 6×10^5 to 7×10^5 cells per well in two ml growth medium (b) and incubate the plates at 37°C in a humidified atmosphere containing 5 % CO_2.
- Wash the monolayers twice with phosphate-buffered saline (a) before use in the assay.

PREPARATION OF TEST SAMPLES AND STANDARD REFERENCE SERA

(Sera to be used in the assay should be heated at 56°C for 30 min.)

- Prepare three fold serial dilutions of the sample to be assayed, in Eagle's medium buffered with Hepes (c) starting at the dilution 1:10
- Dilute in the same way a standard positive reference serum having a significant anti rotavirus titre
- Dilute a negative reference serum 1:10

PERFORMANCE OF THE ASSAY

- Mix one volume of each dilution with one volume of a rotavirus suspension (Thiverval bovine-rotavirus strain ; ref. R. L'Haridon and R. Scherrer 1976) containing 1000 to 1500 plaque-forming-units per ml.
- Incubate for one hour at 37°C
- Inoculate (in duplicate) 0.2 ml of the virus-sample mixtures onto monolayers of MA 104 cells and incubate for 1.5 hour at 37°C with gentle rocking of the plates
- Remove the inoculum and wash the monolayers twice with PBS (a)
- Add two ml agarose - overlay (d) per well and incubate for 4 days at 37°C

- Add a second, two ml agarose-neutral red-overlay (e)
- Cover the plate with aluminium foil and incubate for an additional 4 to 5 hours at 37°C. (plaques having a diameter of 0.5 up to 2.5 mm will be clearly visible)

Reading the results

- Score the number of plaques and express the neutralization titre of a sample as the reciprocal of the dilution causing a 50 % reduction of the number of plaques.

INGREDIENTS

(a) PHOSPHATE BUFFERED SALINE (PBS) pH 7.4

NaCl	8.0 g
KH_2PO_4	0.2 g
Na_2HPO_4; 12 H_2O	2.9 g
KCl	0.2 g
H_2O	A.D. 1000 ml

(b) GROWTH MEDIUM

Eagle's basal medium with Earle's salts (code MBE 0011, Laboratoires Eurobio - 75 Paris, France)

containing :

$NaHCO_3$	0.22 g % (w/v)
Tryptose phosphate	0.16 g % (w/v)
Penicillin	100 IU /ml
Streptomycin	0.1 mg/ml
Foetal calf serum	10 % (v/v)

(c) EAGLE'S MEDIUM-HEPES pH 7.2

MBE 0011 buffered with 20 mM Hepes (N-2 hydroxiethylpiperazine-N'-2-ethanesulfonic acid)

(d) AGAROSE-OVERLAY

MBE 0011 containing :

$NaHCO_3$	26 mM
Tryptose phosphate	0.16 g % (w/v)
Trypsine	0.0017 U/ml
Penicillin	100 IU/ml
Streptomycin	0.1 mg/ml
Agarose	0.6 g % (w/v)

(e)   AGAROSE-NEUTRAL RED-OVERLAY

MBE 0011 buffered with 0.16 M Tris

containing :

Neutral red	0.01 g % (w/v)
Agarose	0.6 g % (w/v)

REFERENCE

L'Haridon, R. and Scherrer, R. : Culture in vitro du rotavirus associé
    aux diarrhées néonatales du veau. Ann. Rech. Vét. 7 (4) : 373-381,
    1976.

MANUAL VI

DETECTION OF BOVINE ENTERITIC CORONAVIRUS (BECV) IN HRT 18 CELLS

Réf. J. Laporte, P. Bobulesco et Françoise Rossi
Une lignée cellulaire particulièrement sensible à la réplication
du coronavirus entéritique bovin : les cellules HRT 18.
C.R. Acad. Sci. Paris 1980, 290 : 623-626.
INRA, Station de Virologie et d'Immunologie, 78850 Thiverval-Grignon, F.

1. PREPARATION OF FAECAL EXTRACTS

- Homogenize one volume of faeces in three volumes of water
- Clarify by low speed centrifugation (2000 g for 20 min at 4°C)
- Use the supernatant diluted 1/10 in RPMI 1640 medium containing 2 % foetal calf serum (FCS), in the test.

2. HRT 18 CELL CULTURE

These Human Rectal Tumor cells were isolated by Tompkins et al. 1974 (J. Natl. Cancer Inst. 52, 1101) ; they are grown as monolayers.

- Confluent cell monolayers in 75 cm^2 are washed with 10 ml PBS and cells dispersed with 1 ml of 0.25 % trypsine + 0.08 % EDTA in PBS ; after addition of 20 ml RPMI medium, cells are centrifuged (700 g, 5 min, room temperature)
- Cell pellet is resuspended in 10 ml 20 % FCS RPMI medium and counted ; Flasks or plates are seeded with 2 x 10^5 cells/cm^2 and incubated at 37°C (plates or petri dishes in a CO_2 incubator)
- Transfer every 4 or 5 days
- If cells are to be infected, change the medium on day 4 after trypsinization (2 % FCS RPMI : maintenance medium).

3. BOVINE ENTERITIC CORONAVIRUS DETECTION

- Infect 6 to 7 day old HRT 18 monolayers prepared in disposable tissue culture plates (Costar 6 wells) with 0.5 ml of the faecal extract in triplicate. Incubate for 1 hr at 37°C in a CO_2 incubator with gentle rocking of the plates.
- Remove the inoculum and wash the cells twice with PBS
- Add 2 ml of 2 % FCS RPMI medium / well and incubate 3 days in a CO_2 incubator at 37°C.

By that time the supernatants of the 3 wells infected with the same
inoculum are pooled ; cells of 1 out of the 3 identical wells are
scraped with a rubber policeman and mixed to the homologous supernatant pool. This cell suspension is kept at - 70°C for the next
passage.
- Cells of the 2 other wells are fixed and stained by indirect
  immunofluorescence technique to visualize infected cells
  Comment : Usually 1 or 2 blind passages are necessary before seeing
  specific fluorescent cells in the monolayer.

4. INDIRECT IMMUNOFLUORESCENCE TECHNIQUE
- Cells are washed twice with cold (4°C) PBS.
- Add 1 ml of cold ethanol (-20°C)/ well, incubate plates for at least
  20 min. at - 20°C.
- Pour out ethanol and dry the plates at 37°C.
- Add 0.5 ml of a 1/300 dilution in PBS of antibovine enteritic corona-
  virus serum and incubate at 37°C for 45 min.
- Wash 5 times with tap water
- Add 0.5 ml of fluorescent anti-rabbit Ig sheep immunoglobulins and
  incubate at 37°C for 30 min.
- Wash 5 times with tap water
- Observe in UV light under the microscope.

5. REAGENTS
. RPMI medium
RPMI 1640 Eutroph medium,* buffered with NaHCO3 (2.0 g/liter) containing
Penicillin 100 U/ml and Streptomycin 0.1 mg/ml
. Anti bovine enteric coronavirus serum
The antiserum was obtained from a rabbit inoculated by subcutaneous
injection of purified BECV in complete Freund's adjuvant. The rabbit
was reinoculated intraveneously two months later with purified virus
alone. The anti coronavirus activity of the serum was checked every two
days by the hemagglutination inhibition test and the rabbit bled 6 to
8 days after the second injection.
. Fluorescent anti rabbit Ig
The conjugate is a commercially available reagent prepared in sheep
(Institut Pasteur Production, Code 74561). The conjugate is diluted
1/200 in PBS for use in the test.

* RPM 1640 Eurobio Paris France.

ELISA FOR THE DETECTION OF BOVINE ROTAVIRUS ANTIGENS IN FAECES

Laboratory manual of the Central Veterinary Institute, Virology Department, 8221 RA Lelystad, The Netherlands.

Reference: Ellens, D.J. and P.W. de Leeuw: Enzyme-linked immunosorbent assay for diagnosis of rotavirus infections in calves. J. clin. Microbiol. 6, 530-532, 1977.

PRINCIPLE OF THE ASSAY

A polystyrene solid phase is coated with antibodies directed against bovine-rotavirus antigens. Upon addition of a faecal extract, rotavirus antigens (if present) will be trapped by specific antibodies covalently linked to the enzyme peroxidase (conjugate). The bound conjugate is visualized through addition of a chromogenic substrate. Specificity of the reaction is checked by blocking the conjugate reaction with a specific anti-rotavirus serum.

MATERIALS AND EQUIPMENT USED

a) equipment

- Polystyrene microtiter plates (Cooke Engeneering, M129-A-E).
- Multichannel pipets + disposable tips.
- Transparent adhesive tape.
- Mechanical vibrators.
- Microtiter plate washer.
- Incubator 37°C.
- Rotator.
- Titertek$^{(R)}$ Multiskan ELISA reader.

b) reagents

- Anti-bovine rotavirus IgG.
- Carbonate-bicarbonate buffer, 0.05 M, pH 9.6.
- Faecal homogenates.
- Standard rotavirus antigen.
- ELISA buffer.
- Conjugate buffer.
- Anti-bovine rotavirus peroxidase conjugate.
- 5-amino-salicylic acid (5-AS) substrate solution.
- Anti-bovine rotavirus blocking serum.

PREPARATION OF BOVINE ANTI-BOVINE ROTAVIRUS (Ba-ROTA) SERUM

- Inoculate a new-born colostrum-deprived SPF or a gnotobiotic calf orally with attenuated or virulent bovine rotavirus.
- Thirty days later inject the calf intramuscularly with 2 ml of purified bovine rotavirus ($\geq 2.10^9$ part./ml), emulsified in complete Freund's adjuvant.
- Repeat the intramuscular injection after 20 days; use incomplete instead of complete Freund's adjuvant.
- Bleed the calf 2-3 weeks after the last injection. Store the serum at -20°C.

SEPARATION OF IgG FROM THE BOVINE ANTI-BOVINE ROTAVIRUS (Ba-ROTA) SERUM

- Add by drops a saturated ammonium sulphate solution to an equal volume (7 ml) of Ba-rota serum of room temperature, which is kept in constant agitation. Let is stand for 8 h at 4°C.
- Collect the precipitate by centrifugation at 1,000 g for 30 min at 4°C.
- Dissolve the pellet in 2 ml of 0.0175 M phosphate buffer, pH 6.3, and dialyse overnight against the same buffer.
- Clarify the solution by centrifugation at 1,000 g for 10 min.
- Apply the sample to a DEAE cellulose column (30 x 1.5 cm) equilibrated against 0.0175 M phosphate buffer, pH 6.3.
- Elute with 0.0175 M phosphate buffer, pH 6.3 and concentrate IgG containing fractions by ammoniumsulphate precipitation.
- Dialyse against 0.15 M NaCl and adjust the IgG concentration to 8 mg/ml.

PREPARATION OF PEROXIDASE CONJUGATED Ba-ROTA IgG ACCORDING TO WILSON AND NAKANE (REF.1)

- Dissolve 8 mg horseradish peroxidase (HRP) (Boehringer, grade I) in 2 ml of distilled water.
- Add 0.4 ml 0.1 M sodium periodate $NaIO_4$ in 0.02 M sodium acetate buffer pH 4.4 and incubate for 20 min at room temperature under constant agitation.
- Dialyse against 1 mM sodium acetate buffer pH 4.4, overnight, 4°C.
- Dialyse 2 ml Ba-rota IgG (8 mg/ml) against 0.01 M carbonate-bicarbonate buffer, pH 9.5.
- Adjust the $HRP-NaIO_4$ solution to pH 9.0 with 0.2 M carbonate-bicarbonate buffer, pH 9.5.
- Add the dialysed Ba-rota IgG solution (2 ml) and incubate for 2 h at room temperature.

- Add 0.2 ml of a freshly prepared solution of sodium borohydride ($NaBH_4$) in distilled water and let it stand for 2 h at room temperature.
- Remove non-conjugated peroxidase by precipitation of the conjugate by adding an equal volume of a saturated ammonium sulphate solution (constant agitation, $4^{o}C$, 90 min).
- Wash the precipitate twice with cold ($4^{o}C$) 50% saturated ammonium sulphate solution, dissolve it in 1 ml demineralized water and dialyse against PBS, pH 7.2.
- Add an equal volume of glycerol and store at $-20^{o}C$.

PREPARATION OF THE 5-AS SUBSTRATE SOLUTION (REF.2).

N.B. This procedure is essential to obtain low background values in the test.

- Dissolve 18 g sodium disulphite ($Na_2S_2O_5$, Merck) and 20 g 5-AS (2-hydroxy benzoïc acid, Merck) in 4 litre demineralized water of 80°-$90^{o}C$.
- Add 2 g of charcoal and stir for 2 min at 80°-$90^{o}C$.
- Remove the charcoal by filtration and cool-down the filtrate rapidly to $4^{o}C$.
- Collect the white precipitate by vacuum filtration through filter paper in a Büchner funnel and wash the precipitate twice with 100 ml demineralized water ($4^{o}C$).
- Dry the 5-AS powder in the dark at room temperature.
- Dissolve 1 g of the purified 5-AS in one litre substrate buffer, pH 6.8. After the addition of 5-AS the pH of the 5-AS solution should be 5.9 (if not adjust).
- Distribute in 10 to 50 ml volumes and store at $-20^{o}C$.
- Prior to use an appropriate volume of the 5-AS solution is thawed, minute precipitates if present are dissolved at $37^{o}C$, and one tenth of the volume of a freshly prepared hydrogen peroxide solution (0.05%) is added.

COATING THE PLATES

- Dilute Ba-rota IgG in carbonate-bicarbonate buffer 0.05 M pH 9.6 to the optimal[1] concentration.
- Apply 100 µl of appropriately diluted Ba-rota IgG solution to the wells and cover with tape.
- Incubate for 18 h at $37^{o}C$ while the plates are rotating at an angle of $45^{o}C$.
- Freeze and store at $-20^{o}C$ for up to two months.

PREPARATION OF FAECAL HOMOGENATES AND STANDARD ANTIGEN

Faecal homogenates

- Apply one g of faeces, 4 ml of ELISA buffer and about 7 glass-beads to a
  7 ml glass vial (can be frozen and stored at -20°C).
- Before testing, homogenize by shaking for one h at room temperature.

Standard antigen

- Homogenize one volume of diarrhoeic faeces of an orally infected SPF calf
  in four volumes of PBS.
- Clarify by centrifugation for 30 min at 1,000 g.
- Add an equal volume of Arklone $^{(R)}$ (I.C.I., U.K.) to the supernatant and
  treat the mixture ultrasonically (3 times, 5 sec, 4°C).
- Separate the phases by centrifugation for 30 min at 1,000 g.
  (Repeat the Arklone and sonification procedure with the water phase,
  if it is too viscous).
- Titrate the water phase in the ELISA; determine and express the concentration of rotavirus antigens in ELISA units (EU). One EU is that dilution giving a P/N value of 3.0.

PERFORMANCE OF THE ASSAY

- Thaw the coated microtiter plate and shower three times with demineralized water containing 0.05% Tween 80.
- Fill the wells of rows 1 and 2 with 100 µl volumes of PBS. Apply 100 µl
  volumes of a two-fold serial dilution of 32 EU standard rotavirus antigen to the wells of rows 3 and 4. Apply, in duplicate, 100 µl volumes
  of 32 faecal homogenates to the remaining 64 wells. Cover with tape.
- Incubate for 18 h at 4°C.
- Shower six times with demineralized water containing 0.05% Tween 80.
- Apply 100 µl volumes of PBS to the wells of the odd-numbered rows, and
  100 µl volumes of appropriately [2)] diluted blocking serum to the wells
  of the even-numbered rows. Cover with tape.
- Incubate for one h at 37°C while the plates are rotating at an angle of
  45°.
- Shower three times with demineralized water containing 0.05% Tween 80.
- Fill the wells of the plate with 100 µl volumes of conjugate buffer
  and an optimal[3)] concentration of anti-bovine rotavirus peroxidase con-
  jugate. Cover with tape.
- Incubate for one h at 37°C.
- Shower four times with demineralized water containing 0.05% Tween 80.
- Fill the wells of the plate with 100 µl volumes of the 5-AS substrate

solution, shake for 10 min and cover with tape.

- Read the test between 3 and 24 h.

READING AND INTERPRETATION

With the naked eye

- Read the colour of the well of the standard rotavirus antigen titration that contains one EU rotavirus antigen.
- Score samples positive that have a colour that is equal to, or more intense than, the colour of the "1 EU" well, and that are blocked by the blocking serum.

With the Titertek ^{R} Multiskan ELISA reader at 450 nm

- Add 100 µl volumes of water to all wells of the plate and shake for 10 min.
- Blanking: enter the values of the blanks (row 1 or 2) into the memory of the instrument.
- Measuring: measure the absorbance at 450 nm of all wells.
- Read the absorbance value of the well of the standard rotavirus antigen titration that contains one EU rotavirus antigen.
- Set the matrix range at ten times the absorbance value of the "1 EU" well.
- Start matrix measuring.
- Score samples positive with matrix values ≥ 1 and that are blocked for $\geq 50\%$.

FOOTNOTES

1) The optimal concentration of Ba-rota IgG for coating should be determined by checkerboard titration:

- Coat a microtiter plate by applying two-fold serial dilutions of Ba-rota IgG in 0.05 M carbonate-bicarbonate buffer pH 9.6 to the wells of rows A-H.
- Shower three times with 0.05% Tween 80.
- Apply two-fold serial dilutions of 32 EU standard rotavirus antigen to the wells of rows 3-12. Fill the wells of rows 1 and 2 with 100 µl volumes of PBS.
- Proceed the ELISA in the normal way.
- The optimal Ba-rota IgG dilution for coating is that dilution which will give positive/negative (P/N) values ≥ 3 with the highest dilution of antigen.

2) Appropriately diluted blocking serum: minimal amount of serum blocking for 90% 32 EU of standard rotavirus antigen.

3) The optimal concentration of Ba-rota-peroxidase conjugate should be determined by checkerboard titration:
- Thaw a coated microtiter plate and shower three times with demineralized water containing 0.05% Tween 80.
- Apply 100 µl volumes of two-fold serial dilutions of 32 EU standard rotavirus antigen to the wells of rows 3-12 and fill the wells of rows 1 and 2 with 100 µl volumes of PBS. Cover with tape.
- Incubate for 18 h at 4°C.
- Shower three times with demineralized water containing 0.05% Tween 80.
- Apply 100 µl volumes of two-fold serial dilutions of the Ba-rota-peroxidase conjugate to the wells of rows A-H and cover the plate with tape.
- Proceed the ELISA in the normal way.
- The optimal Ba-rota-peroxidase conjugate dilution is that dilution which gives P/N values ≥3 with the highest dilution of antigen.

BUFFER SOLUTIONS

Phosphate-buffered saline(PBS), pH 7.2

Sodium chloride (NaCl)	8.0 g	(136.7 mM)
Potassium chloride (KCl)	0.2 g	(2.7 mM)
Disodium hydrogen phosphate ($Na_2HPO_4 \cdot 2H_2O$)	1.44 g	(8.1 mM)
Potassium dihydrogen phosphate (KH_2PO_4)	0.2 g	(1.5 mM)
Demineralized water to	1000 ml	

Stock solutions for phosphate buffers

A. 0.1 M solution of potassium dihydrogen phosphate,
   13.61 g KH_2PO_4 in 1000 ml.
B. 0.1 M solution of disodium hydrogen phosphate,
   17.80 g $Na_2HPO_4 \cdot 2H_2O$ in 1000 ml.
- 0.1 M phosphate buffer, pH 6.8. Adjust the pH of solution A to pH 6.8 with solution B (approximately 510 ml of A and 490 ml of B).
- 0.0175 M phosphate buffer, pH 6.3. Adjust the pH of solution A to pH 6.3 with solution B (about 773 ml of A and 227 ml of B) and dilute 1: 4.71 (4710 ml distilled water to 1000 ml buffer).

Acetate buffer 0.02 M, pH 4.4

A. 0.02 M solution of acetic acid,

1.18 ml acetic acid (96%, d = 1.06 g/ml) in 1000 ml

B. 0.02 M solution of sodium acetate,

1.64 g $C_2H_3O_2Na$ in 1000 ml.

Adjust the pH of solution A to pH 4.4 with solution B (about 305 ml A and 195 ml B).

HAEMADSORPTION - ELUTION - HAEMAGGLUTINATION ASSAY (HEHA) FOR THE
DETECTION OF BOVINE CORONAVIRUS ANTIGENS IN FAECES

Laboratory manual of the Central Veterinary Institute, Virology Department,
39 Houtribweg, 8221 RA Lelystad, The Netherlands.

Reference: J.A.M. van Balken, P.W. de Leeuw, D.J. Ellens and P.J. Straver:
Detection of coronavirus in calf faeces with a haemadsorption - elution -
haemagglutination assay (HEHA). Vet. Microbiol. 3, 205-211, 1978/1979.

PRINCIPLE OF THE ASSAY

The Haemadsorption - Elution - Haemagglutination Assay is based on
the observation that the haemagglutinating activity of bovine coronavirus
present in faecal samples is temperature-dependent. The method consists of
adsorption of the virus onto mouse erythrocytes at $4^{O}C$, removal of unadsorbed material and elution of adsorbed viral material at $37^{O}C$. The eluate
is then used in a haemagglutination test. Specificity of the reaction is
checked by a blocking assay.

1. PREPARATION OF FAECAL EXTRACTS (AND STANDARD ANTIGEN)

- Homogenize one volume of faeces in four volumes of PBS (pH 7.2).
- Clarify by low speed centrifugation (10 min, 1,500 g).
- Use the supernatant fluid in the test.

2. COLLECTION OF WHOLE MOUSE BLOOD

- Anaesthetize adult female mice with chloroform.
- Collect whole mouse blood by heart puncture.
- Mix the blood with an equal volume of an Alsever dextrose solution.
- Centrifuge at low speed (10 min, 200 g).
- Wash the red blood cells several times with PBS until the supernatant
  fluid is clear.

3. ASSAY PROPER

3.1. Haemadsorption

- Mix a 40% suspension of mouse erythrocytes in PBS pH 7.2 with an equal
  volume (0.5 ml) of a faecal extract.
- Incubate for 1 h at $4^{O}C$.
- Centrifuge at low speed (10 min, 200 g).
- Wash the erythrocytes twice with 4.5 ml of PBS of $4^{O}C$.

3.2. Elution

- Add 1 ml of warm PBS (37°C) and mix gently.
- Incubate for 1 h at 37°C.
- Centrifuge at low speed and use the supernatant (eluate) in the haem-agglutination assay.

3.3 Haemagglutination assay

- Prepare two-fold serial dilutions of the supernatant in a microtiter plate, using PBS with 0.2% bovine serum albumin as the diluent (PBS-BSA).
- Add an equal volume (25 μl) of a 1% mouse erythrocyte suspension in PBS-BSA and mix on a mechanical shaker for 5 min.
- Incubate for 90 min at 4°C.
- Read the test with the naked eye.
- Express the HEHA-titres as the reciprocal of the highest antigen dilution showing complete haemagglutination.

4. HAEMAGGLUTINATION INHIBITION (CONFIRMATION) TEST

4.1. Pre-treatment of positive and negative reference sera.

- Inactivate the sera at 56°C for 30 min.
- Mix the sera with equal volumes of 25% Kaolin in PBS and incubate with occasional stirring at room temperature for 45 min.
- Clarify by low speed centrifugation (20 min, 1,000 g).
- Mix the treated serum with an equal volume of a 10% mouse erythrocyte suspension in PBS.
- Incubate for 60 min at 4°C, stir every 10 min.
- Clarify by low speed centrifugation (10 min, 200 g).
- Use the supernatant in the confirmation test.
- Store the treated reference sera in small volumes at -20°C.

4.2. Test proper

- Dilute the eluate of the test samples to contain eight haemagglutinating units in 25 μl.
- Mix with equal volumes of 1:8 in PBS-BSA diluted positive and negative (pre-treated) reference sera.
- Incubate for 45 min at room temperature.
- Add 25 μl of a 1% mouse erythrocyte suspension in PBS-BSA.
- Incubate for 90 min at 4°C and read the test.

  The haemagglutinating activity of a test sample is considered corona-virus specific if complete blocking occurs in the presence of the posi-tive serum, but not in the presence of the negative serum.

5. INGREDIENTS

(Unless stated otherwise, analytical grade chemicals from Merck).

5.1. PBS pH 7.2:

8.0 g NaCl		0.14 M
0.2 g KCl		2.7 mM
1.44 g $Na_2HPO_4 \cdot 2H_2O$		8.1 mM
0.2 g KH_2PO_4		1.5 mM
H_2O	ad	1000 ml

5.2. Alsever-dextrose solution pH 6.1:

20.5 g $C_6H_{12}O_6$		0.11 M	(Brocasef, Deventer, The Netherlands)
8.0 g $C_6H_5Na_3O_7 \cdot 2H_2O$		27.2 mM	
4.2 g NaCl		71.9 mM	
6.01 g $C_6H_8O_7 \cdot H_2O$		28.6 mM	
H_2O	ad	1000 ml	

Sterilize for 15 min at 110°C.

5.3. Kaolin

- Prepare a 25% suspension of Kaolin (Brocasef, Deventer, The Netherlands) in 5N hydrochloric acid, shake and centrifuge (10 min, 1,000 g).
- Wash three times with PBS, each time followed by centrifugation.
- Sterilize a 25% suspension in PBS for 1 h at 121°C and store it at 4°C.

5.4. Reference sera

A reference antiserum against bovine coronavirus was prepared in a 19-day-old SPF calf deprived of colostrum. The calf was inoculated orally with a British isolate and subsequently hyperimmunized with the same strain multiplied in bovine trachea organ cultures. The virus was pelleted from the culture medium at 250,000 g for 30 min, resuspended in PBS, pH 7.2, and emulsified in an equal volume of incomplete Freund's adjuvant. Two ml of this emulsion were injected intramuscularly at 19 and again at 23 weeks of age. Blood was withdrawn 10 days after the last injection.

Pre-serum obtained from the same calf was used as the reference negative serum.

IMMUNOELECTROOSMOPHORESIS (IEOP) FOR THE DETECTION OF BOVINE ROTAVIRUS
ANTIGEN IN FAECES

Two procedures are given in this manual. Procedure A or Procedure B
should be followed throughout.

PROCEDURE A

Laboratory manual of the Central Veterinary Institute, Virology Department,
39 Houtribweg, 8221 RA Lelystad, The Netherlands.

PROCEDURE B

Laboratory manual of the Institute of Medical Microbiology, University
of Copenhagen, Department of Clinical Virology, 22 Juliane Maries Vej,
EK-2100 Copenhagen Ø, Denmark.

REFERENCES

A: Tufvesson, B. and Johnsson, T.: Immunoelectroosmophoresis for detection
    of reo-like virus: methodology and comparison with electron micro-
    scopy. Acta Path. Microbiol. Scand. Sect. B 84, 225-228, 1976.
A: Hopkins, T. and Das, P.C.: Improved sensitivity of the electrophoresis
    method by tannic acid for detection of Australia antigen. J. clin.
    Path. 25, 832-833, 1972.
B: Grauballe, P.C., Genner, J., Meyling, A. and Hornsleth, A.: Rapid
    diagnosis of rotavirus infections: comparison of electron microscopy
    and immunoelectroosmophoresis for the detection of rotavirus in human
    infantile gastroenteritis. J. gen. Virol. 35, 203-218, 1977.

PRINCIPLE OF THE ASSAY

A + B:

In IEOP, immunoprecipitates are formed in agarose gels between wells
containing antibodies to rotavirus (anodic wells) and wells containing
rotavirus antigens (cathodic wells). This is achieved when an agarose with
suitable electroendosmosis and a buffer with suitable pH are used for
electrophoresis.

1. MATERIALS AND EQUIPMENT

1.1. Equipment

Electrophoresis chamber (Gelman) (A + B)

Power supply for 500 V (Gelman) (A + B)

Frames for 6 glass slides (A)

Frame holders (A)

Immunoleveling table (A + B)

Microporous wicks (A)

10 x 10 cm filter paper (Whatman No 1) (B)

Glass slides (25 mm x 75 mm) stored in 70% ethanol (A)

10 x 10 cm x 1 mm glass plates (B)

Trough (A) and wells punch set (A + B)

Dark-ground viewer (A)

1.2.Materials

Tank buffer (A + B)

Agarose (A + B)

Anti-bovine rotavirus globulins (A + B)

Standard rotavirus antigen (A + B)

Tannic acid solution (A)

Coomassie brilliant blue staining solution (A + B)

Destaining solution (A + B)

Normal rabbit immunoglobulin (B)

2. PREPARATION OF RABBIT ANTI-BOVINE ROTAVIRUS (RA ROTA) SERUM

2.1. (A)

- Inject the rabbit intramuscularly with 4 x 0.5 ml bovine rotavirus
  purified in a sucrose gradient ($\geqslant 2.10^9$ part./ml) and emulsified in
  complete Freund's adjuvant.

- Repeat the injection after twenty days and use incomplete instead of
  complete Freund's adjuvant.

- Bleed the rabbit 2-3 weeks after the last injection.

- Store the serum at -20°C.

2.2. (B)

   The antiserum is prepared by inoculation of immunoprecipitates obtained by crossed immunoelectrophoresis of purified human rotavirus against
rabbit antibodies as described in: P.C. Grauballe, A. Meyling and J. Genner:
Immunoelectrophoretic studies of rotaviruses: Preparation of rabbit antibodies to immunoprecipitates of human rotavirus and their use for identification of specific and common antigens of human and bovine rotavirus.
In: Viral Enteritis, INSERM Symposia Series, Vol. 90. F. Bricout and
R. Sherrer (eds.) pp. 413-427, 1979.

3. SEPARATION OF THE GLOBULIN FRACTION FROM THE RA ROTA SERUM BY THE CAP-
RYLIC ACID METHOD

3.1. (A)

- Adjust the Ra Rota serum to pH 4.80 with acetate buffer, pH 4.0.
- Add by drops 0.68 g caprylic acid (d = 0.91 g/ml) per 10 ml of serum and keep the mixture in constant agitation.
- Stir vigorously for 30 min at room temperature.
- Clarify by centrifugation (10 min, 1,500 g).
- Dialyse the supernatant (contains IgG of about 90% purity) against tank buffer.
- Store at -20°C in small aliquots.

4. PREPARATION OF FAECAL HOMOGENATES

4.1. (A + B)

- Apply one g of faeces, 4 ml of PBS and about 7 glass-beads to a 7 ml glass vial.
- Store the vials at -20°C.
- Before testing, thaw and homogenize by shaking for one h at room temperature.
- Clarify by centrifugation at 1,000 g for 10 min. Use supernatant in test.

5. PREPARATION OF 0.75% AGAROSE

5.1. (A)

- Dissolve 750 mg agarose in 100 ml tank buffer by heating.
- Sterilize at 120°C for 15 min.
- Place the solution in a water bath of 100°C.

6. PREPARATION OF THE AGAROSE GELS

6.1. (A)

- Place the frames on the leveling table.
- Flame the glass slides and place them on the frames (six slides each).
- Introduce a small amount of 0.75% agarose (100°C) at the junctures of the slides and the frame.
- Pour 10 ml of 0.75% agarose (cooled down to 45°C) on the slides of a frame section to form a uniform layer.
- Let the agarose gellify for 20 min at room temperature.
- Place the frame holders in a humidified container.
- Let the agarose stabilize for one h at 4°C.
- Punch 9 wells and 3 troughs in each slide.
- Remove gel plugs by suction.

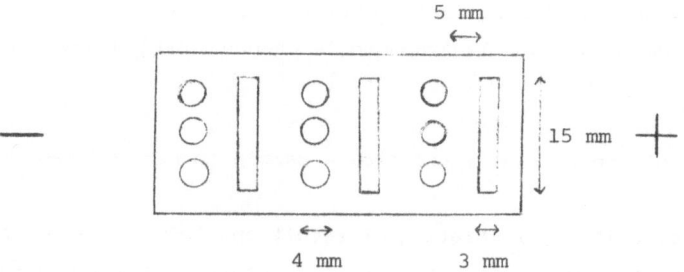

6.2. (B)

- Cover 10 x 10 cm x 1 mm glass plates with 15 ml (50°C) 1% (w/v) melted
  agarose in tank buffer.
- Punch wells (∅ 4 mm) in two rows at a center-to-center distance of 1 cm.
  Two pairs of rows can be cut on each plate if the two rows are staggered.

  1 sample(s) (4-9)

  2 normal rabbit IgG

  3 rabbit anti rotavirus IgG

  10 standard rotavirus

     antigen

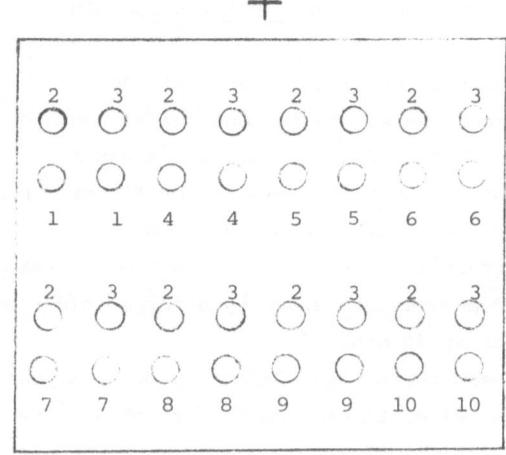

7. IMMUNOELECTROOSMOPHORESIS PROPER

7.1. (A)

- Fill the outer wells with faecal extracts (test samples).
- Fill the middle wells with standard rotavirus antigen.
- Fill the troughs with undiluted caprylic acid treated Ra Rota serum.
- Apply 500 ml of tank buffer to each compartment of the electrophoresis
  chamber.
- Install the frames, equipped with wicks, in the electrophoresis chamber
  in such a way that the troughs are closest to the anode.
- Apply 7 V/cm for 75 min.

- Keep the wicks wet during electrophoresis.
- Remove frames from the electrophoresis chamber and put them in the frame holder.

7.2 (B)

- Add 15 µl of supernatant fluid from a sample to each of two cathodic wells.
- Add 5 µl of 0.1% (IgG) solution of rabbit antibody to one of the anodic wells opposite one of the cathodic wells containing the sample.
- Add 5 µl of 0.1% (IgG) solution of normal rabbit IgG to the other anodic well opposite the remaining cathodic well containing the sample.
- Electrophorese in tank buffer, using filter paper wicks (5 pieces of Whatman No 1 10 x 10 cm in each wick) at 2 V/cm overnight. The plate should be kept at 10-15°C or the electrophoresis should be carried out in a cold room.

8. STAINING OF THE PRECIPITATION LINES

8.1. (A)

Coomassie brilliant blue staining:
- Wash the slides in tank buffer overnight.
- Wash the slides in distilled water for 3 h.
- Cover the slides with moist filter paper and dry overnight at 37°C.
- Moisten filter paper and remove.
- Stain in Coomassie brilliant blue staining solution for 10 min.
- Remove excess stain by a three-fold rinse in destaining solution (3 times 10 min).
- Read the slides. Samples showing a precipitation line at approximately equal distance from the trough and the well are scored positive.

8.2 (A)

Tannic acid staining:
- Wash the slides in tank buffer overnight.
- Stain in a freshly prepared solution of 1% Tannic acid in distilled water for one h.
- Read the slides on the dark-ground viewer. Samples showing a precipitation line at approximately equal distance from the trough and the well are scored positive.

8.3 (B)

- Wash the plate and the wells under running water.
- Cover the gel with a piece of wet filter paper (avoid air bubbles), and

press (10 g/cm^2) the gel in soft tissue for 1 h. Change soft tissue twice during this time.

- Remove the filter paper and dry the gel with a common hair-dryer.
- Stain the gel by immersing the plate in Coomassie brilliant blue solution for 10 min.
- Destain the gel by passing the plate through 3 baths of destainer, 10 min each.
- Dry the destained gel with the hair-dryer and compare the results of a standard rotavirus antigen with the results of the test sample.

9. SOLUTIONS

9.1. (A) Tank buffer, pH 8.6:

Sodium barbital ($C_8H_{11}N_2NaO_3$)   10.30 g 50 mM
Barbital ($C_8H_{12}N_2O_3$)   1.84 g 10 mM
Distilled water to   1000 ml

Dissolve by heating and cool down.

Add 0.41 g calciumlactate ($C_6H_{10}CaO_6 \cdot 5H_2O$) (1.3 mM).

Adjust the pH of the solution to 8.6 with a 37% hydrochloric acid solution.

9.1. (B) Tank buffer, pH 8.6:

56 g Barbital	12 mM	
110 g Tris	36 mM	
2.5 g Ca-lactate	0.45 mM	
H_2O to	25 l	

9.2 (A) Acetate buffer 0.06 M, pH 4.0:

(a) 0.06 M solution of acetic acid.

    3.54 ml acetic acid (96%, d = 1.06 g/ml) in 1000 ml.

(b) 0.06 M solution of sodium acetate.

    4.92 g $C_2H_3O_2Na$ in 1000 ml.

Adjust the pH of solution a to pH 4.0 with solution b (about 100 ml a and 400 ml b).

9.3 (A+B) Phosphate-buffered saline (PBS), pH 7.2:

Sodium chloride (NaCl)	8.0 g	0.14 M
Potassium chloride (KCl)	0.2 g	2.7 mM
Disodium hydrogen phosphate ($Na_2HPO_4 \cdot 2H_2O$)	1.44 g	8.1 mM
Potassium dihydrogen phosphate (KH_2PO_4)	0.2 g	1.5 mM
Distilled water to	1000 ml	

9.4. (A+B) Coomassie brilliant blue staining solution:

Coomassie Brilliant Blue R 250	5 g
Ethanol 96%	450 ml
Glacial acetic acid	100 ml

Magnetic stirring overnight followed by filtration.

Add 450 ml H_2O.

9.5. (A+B) Destaining solution:

Ethanol 96%	450 ml
Glacial acetic acid	100 ml
H_2O	450 ml

10. AGAROSE

10.1. (A) Indubiose A45, l'Industrie Biologique Francaise S.A.

10.2. (B) Litex type HSA, electroendosmosis Mr = -0.13. Litex, 1 Risingevej, DK-2660 Brøndby Strand Denmark. Any other agarose with the same properties may be used.

11. NORMAL RABBIT IMMUNOGLOBULIN

11.1. (B) DAKO-immunoglobulins A/S, 22 Guldborgvej, DK-2000 Copenhagen F, Denmark. Code X 903.

ENZYME-LINKED IMMUNOSORBENT ASSAY (ELISA) FOR THE DETECTION OF ROTAVIRUS
ANTIGENS IN FAECES

Laboratory manual of the Institute of Medical Microbiology, University of
Copenhagen, Department of Clinical Virology, 22 Juliane Maries Vej, DK-2100
Copenhagen Ø, Denmark.

PRINCIPLE OF THE ASSAY

The ELISA technique is based on adsorption of rabbit anti-rotavirus
antibodies (catching Ab) to the surface of wells in microtest plates. After
removal of antibodies not adsorbed, the catching Ab reacts with viral antigens in the faecal suspension. After removal of non-reacting material,
these antigens are detected by antibodies of the same specificity as catching Ab, but conjugated to horseradish peroxidase. After removal of conjugate not bound, the reaction is visualized by adding a solution of ortho-
phenylene-diaminehydrochloride and hydrogenperoxide to the wells.

COATING OF WELLS WITH CATCHING Ab

100 µl of a solution of rabbit anti-rotavirus (human) (3), containing
the concentration in bicarbonate buffer pH 9.6 (5) recommended by the
manufacturer, and an equal amount of normal rabbit IgG (2) are added to
each of two wells in a microtest plate in such manner that later each
specimen can be tested twice with double control.

The plate is incubated at room temperature for 1 h.

WASHING

The contents of the wells are thrown out with force to prevent cross-
contamination and the wells are filled up with washing solution (6) *by immersing the plate in the liquid*. The plate is left for 1 min on the lab.-
table and the procedure is repeated four times. Between each filling the
plate is tapped, upside down, against soft tissue. After this step the
wells may be filled with dilution buffer (7). The plate can then be stored
for at least 4 weeks at +4°C if protected from drying out.

PREPARATION OF FAECAL SAMPLES

One to two g faeces is homogenized in sufficient saline to make a thin
slurry. This suspension is clarified by low speed centrifugation (1,000 g,
10 min). The supernatant is diluted 1:10 in the dilution buffer (7), and
100 µl of the diluted supernatant is added per well (2 test wells plus 2
control wells). Incubate for at least 4 h at room temperature or during the

night at +4°C.

REMOVAL OF FAECAL MATERIAL

The wells are emptied by aid of a water-jet air pump connected to a bottle with chloramine solution and an 8-channeled suction device. The wells are filled with washing solution by multichannel pipette and this procedure is repeated twice. The rest of the washing procedure as in step two.

CONJUGATE

Add the recommended amount of conjugate (4) in 100 µl of dilution buffer (7) per well. Incubate for 30 min at room temperature.

REMOVAL OF UNBOUND CONJUGATE

Wash as described in step two.

STAINING

Add 100 µl of staining buffer (8) per well and empty 1 min later. Add 100 µl of staining solution (9) per well. Incubate for 15 min at room temperature. Stop the reaction by adding 150 µl 2N H_2SO_4/well. Read the results with the naked eye or in a spectrophotometer at 492 nm.

NOTES:

It might be useful to add phenol red, 10 mg/l, to the bicarbonate (5) and the dilution (7) buffers.

If the right microtest plates are used, the assay described will detect less than 1 ng of rotavirus protein. Different microtest plates have been tested. It was found that radiation of the plates was essential and that none of the plates was as sensitive as the Nunc [(R)] plates.

Results read by the naked eye represent approximately 98% of positive specimens read in a spectrophotometer in which the cut-off value is set at A492 0.1 unit and the P/N ratio is $\geq$ 6. This means that a specimen is considered positive for rotavirus if there is a distinct difference between the two test wells and the two control wells as judged by the eye, or if the A492 values of the test wells are $\geq$ 0.1 and the ratio between the A492 values of the test and the control wells is $\geq$ 6. If greater difference than $\pm$ 10% is found between the A492 values of the two test wells the test should be repeated.

INGREDIENTS

If nothing else is stated, all chemicals are analytical grade from Merck.

1. Polystyrene microtest plates: A/S Nunc, 90 Kampstrupvej, DK-4000 Roskilde, Denmark. Code 2-62162.

2. <u>Normal rabbit IgG</u>: DAKO-immunoglobulins A/S, 22 Guldborgvej, DK-2000 Copenhagen F, Denmark. Code X-903.

3. <u>Rabbit anti-rotavirus (human)</u>: DAKO-immunoglobulins A/S. Code B 218.

4. <u>Rabbit anti-rotavirus (human), Peroxidase-conjugated</u>: DAKO-immunoglobulins A/S. Code P 219.

The antiserum is prepared by inoculation of immunoprecipitates obtained by crossed immunoelectrophoresis of purified human rotavirus against rabbit antibodies as described in: P.C. Grauballe, A. Meyling and J. Genner: Immunoelectrophoretic Studies of Rotaviruses: Preparation of Rabbit Antibodies to Immunoprecipitates of Human Rotavirus and Their Use for Identification of Specific and Common Antigens of Human and Bovine Rotavirus. In: Viral Enteritis, INSERM Symposia Series, Vol. 90, Ed. F. Bricout and R. Sherrer, pp. 413-427, 1979.

5. <u>BICARBONATE BUFFER, pH 9.6</u>:

   1.59 g Na_2CO_3 15 mM
   2.93 g $NaHCO_3$ 35 mM
   0.2   g NaN_3 3 mM
   H_2O A.D.   1000 ml
   Store at +4°C for max. 14 days.

6. <u>WASHING SOLUTION, pH 7.2</u>:

   29.20 g NaCl   0.5 M
    0.20 g KCl   2.7 mM
    0.20 g KH_2PO_4 1.5 mM
   1.15 g Na_2HPO_4: $2H_2O$ 6.5 mM
   0.5 ml Tween (R) 20
   H_2O A.D.   1000 ml

7. <u>DILUTION BUFFER, pH 7.2</u>:

   5 g Albumin, bovine (Fraction V, Sigma)
   Washing solution A.D. 1000 ml

8. <u>STAINING BUFFER, pH 5.0</u>:

   Citric acid H_2O 7.3 g   34.7 mM
   Na_2HPO_4 $2H_2O$ 11.86 g   66.7 mM
   H_2O A.D. 1000 ml

9. <u>STAINING SOLUTION, pH 5.0</u>:

   40 mg 1.2-phenylendiamine-dihydrochloride (Fluka or Sigma)
   20 µl 30% H_2O_2
   Staining buffer A.D. 100 ml.
   Stable at +4°C for 24 h if protected from light.

IMMUNODIFFUSION TEST FOR THE DETECTION OF ROTAVIRUS
ANTIGEN IN FAECAL MATERIAL AND GUT HOMOGENATES

E. Van Opdenbosch

Laboratory manual of the National Institute for Veterinary Research
Groeselenberg 99 - 1180 Brussel (Belgium)

1. Materials and equipment used for the test

    1.1. Equipment :

- centrifuge (low speed).

- Ultraturrax (blender)

- magnetic stirrer

- petri-dishes (∅ : 9 cm).

    1.2. Reagents :

- anti-bovine rotavirus serum

- faecal homogenates

- standard rotavirus antigen

- Gelose (Difco) Nobel agar

- merthiolate (Eli Lilly)

- PBS pH 7.2

- TNE buffer pH 8.3

- PEG 6000 (Fluka)

2. Preparation of standard rotavirus antigen

    - Inoculate a confluent monolayer of PK15, secondary calf kidney or testicle cells with rotavirus.

- Freeze-thaw the cells three times after the appearance of a distinct CPE (2-3 days)

- Titrate the suspension and discard if the titre is less than 4×10^5 $TCID_{50}/ml$

- Clarify by low speed centrifugation (600-1,000 g, 30 min)

- Add 600 g of PEG 6000 to ten litres of the supernatant

- Stir overnight at 4° C

- Collect the precipitate by centrifugation (600-1,000 g, 30 min)

- Resuspend the pellet in 100 ml of PBS and add 1 ml of a 1 % solution of merthiolate

- Store the antigen in one ml vials at -20° C

3. Preparation of the bovine anti-rotavirus serum

- Inject a 2-3 months old calf subcutaneously with 10 ml of a cellfree
rotavirus suspension (10^6TCID$_{50}$/ml mixed with 10 ml incomplete Freund's
adjuvant), divided in two sites in the neck.
- Repeat this injection four times at two weeks intervals
- Test the serum for specificity by indirect immunofluorescence (See NIIF
test) two weeks after the last injection. Discard if the titre is less than
3000.

4. Preparation of test samples

- Add two parts of PBS to one part (approximately 5 ml) of faecal ma-
terial or intestinal tissue and mix with an Ultraturrax (0.5 min)
- Clarify by centrifugation (1,000-1,500 g, 30 min)
- Add one ml of PEG 6000 (60 % in PBS) to nine ml of the supernatant
- Incubate at 4° C overnight
- Collect the precipitate by centrifugation (1,000-1,500 g, 15 min)
- Resuspend the pellet in one ml of PBS

5. Preparation of the Gelose

- Make a 5 % w/v solution of Gelose in distilled water and sterilize
at 120° C for 30 min
- Mould the Gelose in pyrex plates to form a 1 cm thick layer
- Cut the Gelose in cubes (1 cm^3)
- Wash the cubes in distilled water twice a day (1 vol. of Gelose in 3 vol.
of water) during one week
- Store the cubes at 4° C
- Add 20 g of Gelose cubes to 80 ml of TNE buffer
- Add PEG 6000 to a final concentration of 3 %
- Add 1 ml of a 0.1 % merthiolate solution
- Liquefy the Gelose cubes at 100° C
- Filter the melted Gelose through a selecta filter (m 597 1/2, Ø 320 mm,
Schleider & Schull) as hot as possible
- Pour 12 ml of the liquid Gelose in a petri dish (Ø : 9 cm) to form a uni-
form layer
- Close the petri dishes when the Gelose is gellified and store (upside
down) at 4° C

6. Assay proper

- Punch just before use four sets of seven wells (Ø : 5 mm) in each
petri dish (fig. 1). The distance between the wells is 5 mm.

- Fill wells nos 1 and 2 with undiluted anti-rotavirus serum
Fill wells nos 4 and 5 with anti-rotavirus serum diluted 1:4
Fill wells nos 3 and 6 with test samples
Fill well no 7 with standard rotavirus antigen
- Incubate at room temperature and read the test after 24-48 h. Samples are scored positive when there is a line of identity with the standard rotavirus antigen

Note :

The sensitivity of the test can be improved by filling the wells twice at six h intervals or by filling the standard antigen and serum wells six h after the sample.

7. Buffer solutions :

7.1 TNE buffer, pH 8.3 :

Tris	0.106M	1.29 g
Sodium chloride (NaCl)	0,189M	11.09 g
Disodium ethylene diaminotetra-acetic acid (Na$_2$EDTA)	0.001M	0.39 g
Distilled water to		1000 ml

7.2 Phosphate buffered saline (PBS), pH 7.2 :

Sodium chloride (NaCl)	0.137M	8.0 g
Potassium chloride (KCl)	0.027M	0.2 g
Disodium hydrogen phosphate (Na$_2$HPO$_4$2H$_2$0)	0.809M	1.44 g
Potassium dihydrogen phosphate (KH$_2$PO$_4$)	0.015M	0.2 g
Distilled water to		1000 ml

Fig. 1

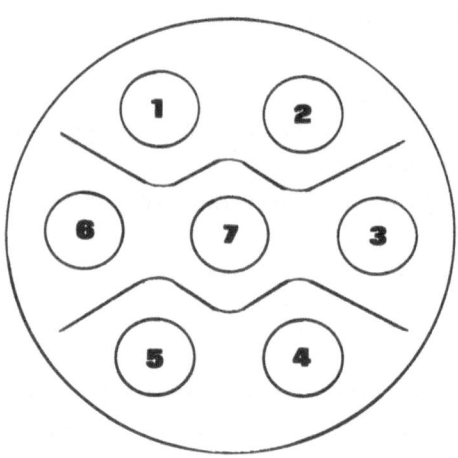

1,2 - undiluted anti-rotavirus serum
4,5 - anti-rotavirus serum, diluted 1:4
3,6 - test samples
7 - standard rotavirus antigen

NEUTRALISATION OF THE INDIRECT IMMUNOFLUORESCENCE TEST (NIIF) FOR THE DETECTION OF ROTA, CORONA AND BVD VIRUS IN BOVINE FAECAL MATERIAL

Emmanuel Van Opdenbosch

Laboratory manual of the National Institute for Veterinary Research

Groeselenberg 99 - B-1180 Brussel (Belgium)

REFERENCE

La neutralisation de l'immunofluorescence indirecte (NIFI) : une technique spécifique et quantitative pour la mise en évidence d'antigènes viraux. G.Wellemans, E.Van Opdenbosch, D.De Kegel, Ann.Méd.Vét.,123, 185-194, 1979.

1. Principe of the test

The test is based on the decrease of the antibody titre of a particular serum which will occur when it is previously incubated with homologous antigen. The test can be used to detect rotavirus, bovine coronavirus or bovine viral diarrhea virus (BVD) in faecal extracts or tissue homogenates. The sera are selected on the basis of their titre in an indirect immunofluorescence (IIF) test.

Cells containing the reference antigen are fixed on a slide. This antigen forms a complex with its corresponding antibody. This complex is evidenced by staining with rabbit anti bovine IgG conjugate. If reference Ab is previously brought in contact with the suspected antigen, a complex will be formed. Therefore, reference antibody is no longer available to react with the infected cells fixed to the slide. Thus there is an inverse relationship between the amount of antigen in the sample and the indirect immunofluorescence titre of the reference serum.

2. Equipment and reagents used in the test

- low speed centrifuge
- Ultraturrax (blender)
- magnetic stirrer
- coated glass slides with ten wells (Glasdekoratie BV, Vigor, Nuland, The Netherlands)
- UV-microscope : indecent leight

Reagents :

- hyperimmune antiserum to bovine rotavirus, bovine coronavirus, and BVD virus.
- standard bovine rotavirus, bovine coronavirus and BVD virus antigen suspensions.
- Rabbit anti-bovine IgG conjugated with fluoresceine isothiocyanate (FITC), free of antibody against the viruses to be detected.

3. Preparation of glass slides with infected cells

- inoculate confluent monolayers of secondary bovine embryo kidney cells with a virus suspension.
- trypsinize the cell cultures when approximately 30 % of the cells is expected to contain antigen detectable by fluorescence (rotavirus one day, bovine coronavirus four days, BVD virus two days).
- wash the cells three times in PBS and resuspend the cells of one Roux flask in 40 ml of PBS.
- put one drop of the cell suspension in each well of the coated glass plates.
- dry the cells at 37° C and fix them in acetone at -20° C during ten min.
- store the slides at -40° C.

4. Selection of reference sera

- carry out an IIF-test (using two-fold dilution steps) with inactivated bovine sera prepared against one viral agent (the serum does not have to be mono-specific).
- discard if the titer is less than 1:810.
- store selected sera in small volumes at -40° C.

5. Preparation of control antigens

- rotavirus and BVD virus : see manual ID-test section A.
- bovine coronavirus : prepare a concentrate of calf rectum found positive for bovine coronavirus by direct immunofluorescence as described in the ID-manual under C.

6. Preparation of test samples

- See ID manual under section C.

7. NIIF test proper

- prepare in each row of a microtiter plate two-fold dilutions of a previously tested hyperimmune serum in PBS (the two highest dilutions should give a negative IIF result).
- add to one row an equal volume of control antigen and to another row an

volume of PBS. The remaining rows are used for the test samples added in equal volumes.

- cover the plate with tape and incubate at 37° C for 12 h.
- put one drop of each of the mixtures in a well of the glass slides containing fixed infected cells and incubate in a humidified atmosphere at 37° C during one h.
- dip the slides in distilled water and wash in PBS at room temperature for one h by magnetic stirring.
- dip again in distilled water, dry the slides, and stain with one drop of an appropriate dilution of a FITC-conjugated anti-bovine IgG preparation.
- incubate the slides in a humidified atmosphere at 37° C for 0.5 h., dip in distilled water, repeat washing in PBS as above, dip in distilled water, and dry.
- add one drop of buffered glycerine pH 9.6 to each well and cover the slides with a cover slip.
- read the results using a UV-microscope.

A negative test is when there is no difference between the titre of the reference serum mixed with the test sample and with PBS. A positive test is when there is four-fold or more reduction of the titre of the reference serum incubated with the test sample as compared to the PBS titre. When a higher titre of the reference serum is found in the presence of the test sample, this means that the test sample contains antibodies directed against the viral antigens present in the fixed cells.

Expression of the antigen titre of a test sample :

reciprocal of the highest positive serum dilution in the presence of PBS
idem in the presence of the test sample

8. Buffers and materials

Carbonate-bicarbonate buffer pH 9.6 :
- $NaHCO_3$ 21 g   0.250 M
- Na_2CO_3 26.5 g   0.250 M
- dissolve in one litre of distilled water.

Buffered glycerine, pH 9.6 :
- glycerine   9 ml
- carbonate-bicarbonate
buffer pH 9.6   1 ml

PEG 6000 : Fluka AG, Buchs, Switserland.

124

IF-TEST IN THE DIAGNOSIS OF VIRAL GASTROENTERITIS IN PIGS

Laboratory manual of the Laboratory for Virology, Faculteit van de Diergeneeskunde, 24 Casinoplein, B9000 Gent, Belgium.

Reference: Pensaert, M.B., Haelterman, E.O. and Burnstein, T.:
Diagnosis of transmissible gastroenteritis in pigs. Can. J. Comp. Med. 32, 556-561, 1968.

INTRODUCTION

For laboratory diagnosis of viral gastroenteritis by means of immunofluorescence, we demand that *living* piglets having diarrhea for less than two days should be brought to the laboratory. This is required because postmortal changes occur very quickly in the small intestinal mucosa and the villi readily loose their epithelial cells. Since the viral antigens are to be detected in those cells, it is of the highest importance that they are still present.

All sections are routinely stained with three specific conjugates, i.e. against TGE virus, rotavirus and the coronavirus-like agent (CVLA).

CONJUGATES

The antiserum against TGE virus was raised in a conventional pig. The antisera against rotavirus and CVLA were raised in SPF pigs. For hyperimmunisation of the pigs, a first oral inoculation was followed by several intramuscular injections of virus emulsified in complete Freund's adjuvant. All these sera were tested for their monovalent specificity before the conjugation with fluorescein isothyocyanate which was performed at the National Institute for Veterinary Research (NIDO-Ukkel).

METHODS

- Two pieces of jejunum (middle and last third) of 0.5 cm length are taken from the pigs immediately after they are killed.
- Gelatin capsules, size 00, are filled with embedding medium for frozen tissue specimens (Tissue-Tek II O.C.T. Compound: Lab-Tek Products). The piece of jejunum is placed in the capsule by means of a small forceps, allowing the embedding medium to penetrate the lumen.
- The capsule is closed and quickly frozen in a dry ice-alcohol bath.
- The frozen capsules are wiped free of alcohol and can be stored in the freezer (-25°C) until further processing.

- Before mounting the embedded tissue on the cryostat specimen-holder, the gelating capsule must be peeled off.
- Sections are cut, 8 μ thick, and collected on fat-free slides.
- The slides are allowed to dry before they are fixed in cold acetone (-20°C) for 20 minutes. Subsequently, they are dried in the freezer for another 10-20 minutes.
- The sections are washed in phosphate buffered saline (PBS) pH 7,2 for 10 minutes and dried in a warm air stream.
- The sections are outlined with a wax pencil (Marktex Tech-Pen, Englewood N.J., USA) and a drop of the appropriate conjugate at the working dilution is put on each section.
- The slides are incubated in a moist chamber at 37°C for 45 minutes.
- The slides are washed in three changes of PBS, 10 minutes each and are immersed in distilled water for 1 minute before drying in a warm air stream.
- The sections are mounted with a coverslip using buffered glycerine (9 parts glycerine, 1 part of PBS) and are examined.
- Positive sections show a clear intracytoplasmic fluorescence in the villous epithelial cells.
- When the processed material originates from living pigs having a diarrhea for less than two days, a negative fluorescence for TGE and CVLA means that those viruses are not involved.
  A negative fluorescence for rotavirus, however, may not be decisive for the absence of the virus since the rotavirus-containing epithelial cells can disappear rather quickly after the onset of the diarrhea.
  The latter point should, however, be investigated further before definite conclusions can be made.

ESCHERICHIA COLI ASSOCIATED WITH NEONATAL DIARRHOEA IN PIGLETS AND CALVES

P.A.M.Guinée[1], W.H.Jansen[1], T.Wadström[2] and R.Sellwood[3]

[1] National Institute of Public Health,

P.O.Box 1,

3720 BA Bilthoven,

The Netherlands.

[2] Department of Bacteriology and Epizootology, College of Veterinary
Medicine, Swedish University of Agricultural Sciences,
Biomedicum, Box 583,
S-751 23 Uppsala,

Sweden.

[3] Biochemistry Department,

Institute for Research on Animal Diseases,

Compton, Berkshire,

England.

CONTENTS

1. Introduction

Enteric disease in man and animals caused by Escherichia coli can be
classified into several forms (Moon, 1974).

a. Oedema disease is an example of the enterotoxaemic form, hitherto found only in pigs.

b. Colisepsis in neonatal calves is an example of the septicaemic form.

c. The invasive form has, until now, only been found as an intestinal disease in humans, and is very similar to shigellosis.

d. Neonatal diarrhoea in piglets and calves are examples of the entero-toxigenic form.

This paper is limited to the enterotoxigenic form in animals.

2. Concept of the pathogenesis of neonatal E.coli enterotoxin-induced diarrhoea.

The E.coli bacteria gain access to the victim by the oral route. The bacteria pass easily through the stomach because stomach pH is still about neutral in the newly-born piglet and reach the small intestine. The enterotoxigenic E.coli overcome the peristalsis of the small intestine and proliferate because they are able to adhere to the wall of the small intestine by means of adhesins. Enterotoxin(s) are thus produced very near to their receptor sites in the intestinal mucosa. They induce the secretion of water and electrolytes into the lumen, resulting in diarrhoea, dehydration and death.

The localization of the E.coli in the small intestine depends on the type of adhesin and the animal host. Strains possessing the adhesin K88 adhere primarily in the anterior small intestine in piglets. Strains possessing the adhesin P987 adhere in the posterior small intestine in piglets. Strains possessing the adhesin K99 adhere in the middle and posterior parts of the small intestine in calves and piglets (Smith and Huggins, 1978).

Although enteropathogenicity seems to be determined by two factors, enterotoxigenicity and adhesion, it is probably an oversimplification to state that these two factors are the only prerequisites for enteropathogenicity.

3. Enterotoxin assay in vivo and in vitro.

The original concept of enterotoxin was based on the detection of a heat-labile enterotoxin in Vibrio cholerae, by means of the ligated gut test (LGT) in rabbits (De and Chatterjee, 1953). In porcine E.coli strains, originally two types of enterotoxin were distinguished (Smith and Gyles, 1970a):

a. LT (labile toxin): is inactivated by heat at 60°C, has a high MW

(> 100 000), is immunogenic, consists of two subunits and cross-reacts with <u>V.cholerae</u> enterotoxin.

b. ST (stable toxin): is not inactivated by heat at 100°C for 15 minutes,
has a low MW (< 20 000) and is non-immunogenic.

Both types of enterotoxin are plasmid controlled (Smith and Halls, 1968).

3.1. In vivo assay of LT and ST

The two types of toxins can be detected in the LGT using pig intestine as well as rabbit intestine. The LGT in pigs of 4-6 weeks, or even
8-12 weeks (Smith and Gyles, 1970b), has become one of the standard tests
for assay of enterotoxin of porcine strains (Smith and Halls, 1967). The
technique is described in manual 3.

Moon and Whipp (1970) described so-called "class II-strains" with
serotypes 0101:K(A)? and 064:K? which were positive in the LGT in pigs
less than 2 weeks old, intermediate in pigs 2-6 weeks and negative in
older pigs. Smith and Linggood (1972) reported that these strains did not
dilate intestinal loops of 4-6 weeks old pigs, but did dilate the intestine of 1-2 days old piglets. Enterotoxins produced by these strains were
found to be of the ST variety. Evans et al. (1973), when studying ST-producing <u>E.coli</u> strains of human origin, found that the response in rabbit
ileal loops was maximal after 6 hours. ST-producing strains of porcine origin have not been tested in this way in the LGT using pig intestine. It
might be worthwhile to do so, because the response to ST in the LGT using
pig intestine after 24 hrs. was found to be poor compared to that of LT
(Guinée and Jansen, 1979b). While a number of in vitro systems for LT-
assay have been developed, ST-assay can only be done by means of an in
vivo system. In addition to the LGT, the suckling mouse test (SMT) has
been used on a large scale. The SMT originally described by Dean et al.
(1972) and standardized by Gianella (1976) was found to be a reliable tool,
but several minor modifications were made in order to improve the practical
value of the test (Guinée and Jansen, 1979b). The principle of the test is
the injection of an ST-preparation into the stomach of suckling mice causing fluid accumulation in the intestinal tract after several hours. Optimal results are dependent on:

1. selection and handling of mice
2. culturing conditions of the suspected bacterial strain
3. recording of the results.

The Suckling Mouse Test (SMT) is described in detail in manual 2.

The SMT is generally considered to be a reliable indicator of ST. However, a few reports indicating the existence of two or more types of ST and incriminating the diagnostic value of the SMT should be mentioned. Burgess et al. (1978) identified two forms of ST in a porcine, atypical strains P16 (serotype 09:K9), STa and STb. The toxins were separated by methanol extraction. STa was methanol soluble, active in the LGT in neonatal piglets of 1 to 3 days old (18 hrs. autopsy) and in the SMT, but inactive in the LGT with pigs of 7-9 weeks. STb was methanol insoluble, active in the LGT with weaned pigs and rabbits, but inactive in the SMT. STb had greater heat stability than STa. Gyles (1979) compared the response of three different tests using ST preparations of several E.coli strains. The tree tests were:

1. LGT in 6-8 week old pigs, autopsy at 16-18 hrs. post operationem
2. LGT in rabbits, autopsy at 6 hrs. post operationem
3. SMT, oral infection instead of intragastric infection.

Two patterns of reaction were observed: the ST preparation elicited a response in all three tests or in the ligated pig intestine only. Apparently there were two kinds of ST in porcine strains (STa and STb). Olssen and Söderlind (1980) distinghuished three types of ST in porcine strains which they designated: "ST pig + mouse", "ST pig" and "ST mouse".

So, neither the SMT nor the LGT in piglets (18 hrs.) seem to indicate ST in all ST^+ strains. A study using LGT in 4-6 week old piglets autopsied after times shorter than 18-24 hrs., in comparison to the LGT in neonatal piglets as well as to the SMT therefore seems to be desirable.

3.2. In vitro assays of LT

LT stimulates the synthesis of 3'5' cyclic adenosine monophosphate (cAMP) (Kantor et al., 1974; Kimberg et al., 1971). The assay test based on this phenomenon was found to be valid, but to have limited practical value only (Guinée and Jansen, 1979b). LT was found to cause the rounding of mouse adrenal tumor Y1 cells (Donta et al., 1973a, 1973b). Also chinese hamster ovary (CHO) cells respond with characteristic morphological changes to LT (Guerrant et al., 1974). More recently, the continuous cell-line of African green monkey kidney (Vero) was found to respond characteristically to LT (Speirs et al., 1977). Moreover, some E.coli strains of human origin were found to produce a cytotoxin that differed from LT and ST. The cytotoxin was toxic for Vero, but not for Y1 and CHO cells and its effect on Vero cells was distinctly different from that of LT (Konowalchuk

et al., 1977). Moreover, Vero cells are simple and economical to maintain
in the laboratory. The Vero cell test may therefore be considered as the
most attractive in vitro test for LT. Vero cells are commercially available (ATCC or Flow) and are easily maintained in medium 199 plus Earle
salts and 5% neonatal calf serum (Flow) in a humidified atmosphere of 5%
CO_2 in air. Vero cells are routinely employed in many diagnostic virologi-
cal laboratories. The recommended procedure for the detection of LT by
means of Vero cells is described in manual 4.

Enterotoxin assay of porcine strains may be summarized as follows:

Entero-toxin	LGT in pigs 4-6 weeks old	LGT in pigs < 2 weeks	SMT	Y1	CHO	Vero
LT	+	+	−	+	+	+
STa	+	+	+	−	−	−
STb	+[1]	+	−	−	−	−

[1] negative according to Smith and Linggood (1972); positive according
to Gyles (1979).

4. Adhesins.

The adhesive properties of E.coli are commonly associated with antigens whcih appear on the surface of the bacterial cell. The term "adhesin"
has been used to describe substances which mediate attachment of organisms
to a surface (Duguid, 1959). Adhesins often associated with E.coli isolated from pigs with diarrhoea are K88 and P987 (Nagy et al., 1976; Sojka,
1965). The adhesin K99 can also be identified on E.coli isolated from pigs
with diarrhoea (Moon et al., 1977) but is more commonly found on the surface of E.coli associated with diarrhoea in calves (Myers and Guinée,
1976; Smith and Linggood, 1972).

These adhesins appear on the surface of the bacterial cell in two
morphologically distinct forms. The K88 and K99 adhesins appear in
electron microscope studies of metal-shadowed specimens as fine, branching,
fibrillar structures of 40-60 Å in diameter (Burrows et al., 1976; Jones,
1972). The P987 adhesin is easily visualized by negative staining techniques and the filaments are long and straight of approximately 70 Å in
diameter and up to 2 μm in length (Isaacson et al., 1977). In this respect
they are very similar to type 1 fimbriae produced by most E.coli strains
(Duguid et al., 1955). All three adhesins are composed of thermolabile

protein: the K88 antigen consists of equal subunits of approximately
25 000 Daltons (Mooi and de Graaf, 1979); the K99 antigen is made up of
subunits of 22 500 and 29 500 Daltons (Isaacson, 1977) and the 987 pilus
antigen has subunits of approximately 22 500 Daltons (Sellwood, unpublished observations). The K88 antigen occurs in at least three distinct serological varieties K88ab, K88ac (Ørskov et al., 1964) and K88ad (Guinée and
Jansen, 1979a) and each is also serologically distinct from the K99 and
P987 adhesins.

These adhesins are coded for in the bacterial cell by plasmids the
transfer of which from a donor to a recipient strain can easily be accomplished by conjugation (Burrows et al., 1976; Ørskov and Ørskov, 1966).
When the K88 plasmid is transferred in this way the ability to ferment
raffinose is also usually transferred. Therefore, K88$^+$ transconjugants can
often be obtained by testing raffinose fermenting transconjugants for the
production of K88 antigen (Guinée and Jansen, 1979a). The expression of
these adhesins is temperature-dependent and they are not expressed when
cultured at 20°C (Isaacson, 1977; Ørskov et al., 1961; Ørskov et al.,
1975).

Type 1 fimbriae also have adhesive properties but there appears to
be an important difference between these structures and the adhesins described. Attachment to a variety of cells mediated by the adhesins K88,
K99 and P987 is not inhibited by D-mannose whereas the adhesive ability
of type 1 fimbriae of many E.coli strains investigated is specifically
inhibited by this sugar. Also pellicle formation in static broth culture
is associated with both type 1 fimbriae and P987 adhesin production. However, this is also inhibited when D-mannose is added to the medium of
type 1 fimbriae-producing organisms (Old et al., 1968). This does not
occur when the P987 E.coli strains are treated in the same way. Moreover,
mannose-sensitive adhesion mediated by type 1 fimbriae has not been shown
to have any importance regarding enteropathogeneity of E.coli strains.

An important consideration in the investigation of the presence of
adhesin is that of the conditions of culturing the organisms. Each of the
adhesins requires different nutrients or conditions for its expression:
1. The K88 antigen is readily synthesized on commercially available
   nutrient media such as nutrient agar or blood agar.
2. The K99 antigen is very discerning in its requirements and is optimally
   produced on minimal media when enriched with IsoVitalex (Minca-Is

medium) (Guinée et al., 1976; Guinée et al., 1977b) or on tryptose
yeast extract agar (TEM-manual 8) (Burrows et al., 1976). It has been
reported also that there is suppression of the K99 plasmid by the
presence of glucose in the medium (Isaacson, 1980).

3. The P987 adhesin should be grown in static broth culture for the
   formation of pellicle production (Isaacson, 1977) or on Slanetz agar
   (Sellwood, unpublished observations, manual 8).

Techniques for the assessment of adhesin production include (a) slide
agglutination tests, (b) haemagglutination and (c) adhesion to intestinal
epithelial cells or brush-borders. However, one should be aware of possible problems when conducting these tests. Slide agglutination tests of
P987 strains cultured directly from faecal swabs on blood agar and Slanetz
agar are subject to many inconsistencies. The reason for this is that
there is phase variation and usually only 10-20% of colonies are piliated.
It is therefore often useful to test for the presence of accompanying
"K" antigens (e.g. K103), the presence of which are stable. The erythrocytes used in haemagglutinating assays should be standardized using
strains of E.coli known to express the antigens. The temperature at which
the test is conducted can also be important as well as the sensitivity
to mannose (Jones and Rutter, 1974). It is also known that the P987 adhesin
does not cause haemagglutination. Adhesion studies must utilize brush-
borders prepared from susceptible animals, either genetically susceptible
as in the case of K88 adherence to pig brush-borders when some pigs do not
have the receptor for the K88 adhesin (Sellwood et al., 1975), or from
animals at the most susceptible age (Runnels et al., 1980). Brush-borders
must also be used from the area of intestine most susceptible to adhesion
when considering the attachment of K99[+] organisms (Sellwood and Lees,
1980). New adhesins are being discovered regularly but no single technique
can be applied for studying their presence and the conditions of the
tests for identifying them vary tremendously. It is only with a wide
approach to the problem, employing more than one technique that the presence of adhesins can be adequately investigated.

Storage of strains in liquid broth media supplemented with 15% glycerol at -70°C gives good stability of the enterotoxin properties as well
as of the surface adhesins (K88, K99, and CFA in human ETEC strains) over
several years of observations time. Storage on Dorset Egg medium (Oxoid)
at 4°C is also a good alternative while freeze drying can give unpredict-

able results in our hands (T.Wadström and A.Faris, unpublished data).

5. Antigenic (serological) properties of E.coli, preparation of antisera and serotyping of E.coli.

The individual isolates of E.coli possess a variety of antigenic determinants. Three surface antigens are currently being used for diagnostic purposes: O, H and K antigens.

a. The O antigen is the specific polysaccharide of the cell-wall lipolysaccharide. It is thermostable i.e. heating at 100°C for 2 hrs., does not alter its serological specificity. Until now, 163 different O antigens (termed O1-O163) have been recognised and established (Establishment of new E.coli antigens (O, H or K) is coordinated by the World Health Organization Collaborative Centre for Reference and Research on Escherichia coli in Copenhagen (dr.Ida and Frits Ørskov).

b. Many E.coli strains are motile due to the presence of flagella. Flagella possess a so-called flagellar or H antigen. It consists of protein and is thermolabile. Fifty five H antigen (H1-H55) have been established.

c. Many E.coli cultures possess a capsular or K antigen. When the E.coli serology was developed in the late forties, Kauffmann used O inagglutinability as a criterium for the presence of a K antigen. Strains which, in the living state, do not react in homologous pure O antiserum (prepared with cultures heated at 100°C or 121°C; see manual 6) were considered to possess a K antigen. In this way, 103 K antigens (K1-K103) were established. All K antigens are inactivated by heating at 100°C for 2 hours, except those of the so-called A variety, which are inactivated by heating at 121°C for 2 hours only. Recent studies by Ørskov et al. (1977) have indicated that only part of the already established K antigens consist of polysaccharide. They have proposed to omit the non-polysaccharide K antigens from the diagnostic system, with the exception of fibrillar antigens such as K88 and K99 (see chapter 4). Of the 103 originally established K antigens 31 will be deleted, including K antigens of porcine strains. The nomenclature of fibrillar antigens may be altered in the near future. We follow this proposal by placing non-polysaccharide, non-fibrillar and non-pili, K antigens between brackets. Some O and K antigens were later found to occur in 2 or 3 serological varieties, for example
O128: O128ab and O128ac
K88: K88ab, K88ac and K88ad.

The results of the analysis of O, K and H antigens (serotyping) are presented as a serotype, for example:

0101:K30:K99:NM (= non-motile)

0149:(K91):K88ac:H19[a]

0101:K-[b]

0101:K?[c]

[a] (K91): no true polysaccharide K antigen, will be deleted from the typing system.

[b] K-: no K antigen.

[c] K?: in the living state the strain does not react in any of the OK antisera, nor in its homologous O antiserum. However, the presence of a capsular polysaccharide has not been proven.

It should be pointed out that, due to the enormous antigenic variety of E.coli, preparation and particularly control on specificity of E.coli antisera is a task for specialised laboratories. The reader is referred to standard textbooks on the subject by Edwards and Ewing (1972) and Sojka (1965).

The choice of techniques to be employed for serotyping of E.coli depends on the question one wishes to answer:

I. to which serotype does a particular strain belong (complete serotyping)?

II. does a particular strain belong to a particular (series of) serotype(s) or does it possess a particular antigen (partial serotyping)?

Recommended methods are outlined in manual 6.

6. Serotypes of E.coli associated with neonatal enterotoxin-induced diarrhoea in piglets and calves.

6.1. Porcine strains

Enterotoxigenic strains found in piglets may be subdivided into four classes. It should be stressed that no strict boundaries between the classes can be drawn.

a. Typical or classical strains (serotypes) in piglets.

b. Strains with bovine serotypes; these strains possess the K99 antigen (adhesin) and are primarily encountered in calves and lambs.

c. Atypical or "class II" strains in piglets (see also part 3 of this chapter).

d. Strains of porcine origin with other serotypes and proven to be enterotoxigenic.

6.1.1. Typical or classical strains of porcine origin

The serotypes listed in Table 1 have been encountered in many strains and many countries. It should be noted that a shift in the prevalence of particular serotypes has been observed. Serotype 0149:(K91):K88ac:H19 is predominant in many countries at this moment.

Table 1. Serotypes of classical porcine enterotoxigenic E.coli strains.

Serotype	W.H.O.Reference Centre standard strain (other designation and literature reference)
08:K87:K88ab:H19	G7
08:K87:K88ac:H19	G205
08:K87:K88ad:H19	(H56; see Guinée and Jansen, 1979a)
0138:(K81):K88ac:H19	G491
0139:K82:H1[*]	E4
0141:(K85ab):K88ab:H4	E68
0141:(K85ac):K88ab:H4	G1108E
0147:(K89):K88ac:H19	G1253
0149:(K91):K88ac:H10	A1
0157:K-:K88ac:H19	A2

[*] Strains with serotype 0139:(K82):H1 are usually non-enterotoxigenic (Söderlind, 1973). However, ST-producing strains have been described recently (Gyles, 1979).

Strains belonging to these serotypes produce ST and/or LT. It should be stressed that strains with these serotypes but devoid of K88 antigen may be encountered in cases of E.coli infections. The majority of such strains produce one or more enterotoxins (Moon et al., 1980; Söderlind, 1973; Söderlind and Möllby, 1979). In such cases, the correlation between serotype (OK-type) and production of enterotoxin(s) is used for the diagnosis.

6.1.2. Strains with bovine serotypes occurring in piglets also

See Table 3.

6.1.3. Atypical or "class II" strains in piglets

These strains are considered to be atypical, because their ST dilates only intestine of newly-born piglets and not that of 4-6 weeks old pigs (Moon and Whip, 1970; Smith and Linggood, 1972). Serotypes of atypical strains are 0101:K? and 064:K?.

6.1.4. Strains of porcine origin with other serotypes and proven to be enterotoxigenic

As already pointed out, prerequisites for enteropathogenicity, production of adhesin and enterotoxin, are plasmid-controlled. It is therefore conceivable that these characters may be disseminated to strains of other serotypes, thus rendering them enteropathogenic. A number of enterotoxigenic strains with non-classical serotypes have been isolated from diseased or succumbed piglets. It is unpredictable whether such strains will remain sporadic (non-endemic) or may become established and eventually replace the now classical serotypes. Careful monitoring of such strains is therefore indicated.

Table 2. Porcine enterotoxigenic E.coli strains with other serotypes.

Serotype	Enterotoxin	Reference
07:K-[a]:H4	LT	1[f], 2[f]
08:K?[b]:K88ac:H19	LT	1
08:K?:K88ad:H19	LT	1, 3[f]
08:K83:H21	LT	1
08:K"200"[c]:H31	LT	1
08:K"422":H14	LT	1
09:K(A)?[d]:K88ad	LT, ST	3
09:K103:P987:NM	ST	4[f], 5[f]
0X46:K103:P987:NM	ST	1, 2
09:K"2347":K88ad:NM	LT, ST	1
016:K83:H20	LT	1
020:K?:K88ac:NM	LT	1
035:K-:H6	LT	1, 2, 6[f]
045:K-:K88ac:H19 or NM	LT	1, 6
054:K-:H21	ST	1
0101:K103:K88ac:NM[e]	LT	
0108:K-:H9	ST	1
0137:K-:NM	LT	1
0142:K-:NM	LT	1

a) K-: no K antigen.
b) K?: in the living state, the strain does not react with any of the established OK antisera nor with its homologous O antiserum. However, the presence of a capsular polysaccharide has not been proven.

c) K"200", K"422" and K"2347" are provisionally designated K antigens
(see Guinée et al., 1977a).
d) K(A)?: see b). Heating at 121°C is required to render the strain
agglutinable with its homologous O antiserum.
e) This strain was received from dr.Pestana de Castro, Sao Paulo, Brasil.
f) Ref. 1: Guinée et al., 1977a.
Ref. 2: Söderlind, 1973.
Ref. 3: Guinée and Jansen, 1979a.
Ref. 4: Guinée and Jansen, 1979b.
Ref. 5: Isaacson et al., 1977.
Ref. 6: Sojka, 1965.

6.2. Bovine strains

All enterotoxigenic strains of bovine origin produce ST and K99
(Guinée and Jansen, 1979b). They are listed in Table 3. The diagnosis of
enterotoxin-induced diarrhoea may therefore be based on the detection of
K99 antigen. Further serotyping has no further diagnostic value.

Table 3. Serotypes of classical bovine enterotoxigenic E.coli strains.

O8:K25:K99	O20:K?:K99
O8:(K85):K99	O101:K28:K99
O9:K30:K99	O101:K30:K99
O9:K35:K99	O101:K(A)?:K99
O9:K(A)?:K99	O101:K-:K99

7. Closing remarks.

The results of antibiotic therapy of neonatal enterotoxin-induced
diarrhoea are increasingly disappointing, mainly because:
1. the disease rapidly leads to death and antibiotic therapy comes too
   late, especially in the newborn piglet.
2. an increasing number of strains have become multiple-resistant due to
   the presence of resistance plasmids.

Therapy with rehydration solutions has been reported to be successful.
For the prevention of enterotoxin-induced diarrhoea in piglets, vaccination of the sows has been reported to be successful. Vaccines either
contain formalin-killed bacteria of several serotypes including the K88
antigen(s) or more or less purified K88 antigen. Although apparently
successful, such vaccines might eventually turn out to be of limited
value, for example because they do not protect against infections with
K99[+] or P987[+] strains. Careful monitoring of enterotoxigenic strains isolated from vaccinated herds is therefore to be recommended, because new

serotypes may come up.

A Veterinary Investigation Centre should be able to recognise the classical porcine and bovine enterotoxigenic serotypes by means of slide agglutination tests. When strains not belonging to such serotypes, but suspected of being enteropathogenic, are encountered, further tests should be done, probably in a more specialised laboratory. It is recommended to test such strains for enterotoxins rather than for serotype. For LT, the Vero test or a LGT using pig intestine is appropriate. For ST, the LGT using pig intestine should be used. Suspected enterotoxigenic strains with non-classical serotypes should be carefully monitored because they might escape the protection provided upon herds by means of vaccination with K88 and K99 antigen-containing vaccines. Serotyping of these strains will be a considerable attribute to the monitoring program. In this way the establishment of new serotypes can be observed. This might have conse- quences for the composition of vaccines as well as for the required availability of diagnostic antisera in the field. Development of more simple and rapid tests for LT testing is underway in several laboratories. Enzyme-linked Immunosorbent assay (ELISA) and a variant called GM_1-ELISA have recently been developed for rapid detection of LT on human entero- toxigenic E.coli (Sack et al., 1980), but there is yet no data in detec- tion of LT in strains from piglets in the literature. Development of a coagglutination method for rapid detection of LT in suspended colonies from primary isolations lysed by EDTA-lysozyme treatment has given very promising results with staphylococci coated with monovalent cholera toxin/ antiserum (Wadström and Rönnberg, in preparation). The recent report on production of antiserum to ST (Lathe et al., 1980) previously reported to be non-antigenic indicates new possibilities to develop also in vitro immunodiagnostic tests for this toxin(s). Such new developments will greatly facilitate and encourage epidemiological studies of enterotoxi- genic E.coli both in veterinary and human medicine.

Other species of enterotoxin-producing organisms among enterobacteria than E.coli have been isolated from humans with acute diarrhoeal disease (Wadström et al., 1976) while only very few reports describe isolation of such organisms from animals. However, a study on experimental diarrhoea in calves recently showed that enterotoxigenic Klebsiella organisms can cause fulminant diarrhoea in this species (Wilcock, 1979). These observa- tions clearly indicate that enterotoxigenic bacteria other than E.coli may have been ignored until recently as an aetiology of neonatal diarrhoea in young animals.

References

Burgess, M.N., Bywater, R.J., Cowley, C.M., Millan, N.A. and Newsome, P.M.: Biological evaluation of a methanol-soluble, heat-stable Escherichia coli enterotoxin in infant mice, pigs, rabbits and calves. Infect. Immun. 21: 526-531, 1978.

Burrows, M.R., Sellwood, R. and Gibbons, R.A.: Haemagglutinating and adhesive properties associated with the K99 antigen of bovine strains of Escherichia coli. J.Gen.Microb. 96: 269-275, 1976.

De, S.N. and Chatterjee, D.N.: An experimental study on the mechanism of action of Vibrio cholerae on the intestinal mucous membrane. J.Path. Bacteriol. 66: 559-562, 1953.

Dean, A., Ching, Y.C., Williams, R.G. and Harden, L.B.: Test for Escherichia coli enterotoxin using infant mice: application in a study of diarrhea in children in Honolulu. J.Infect.Dis. 125: 407-411, 1972.

Donta, S.T., King, M. and Sloper, K.: Induction of steroidogenesis in tissue culture by cholera enterotoxin. Nature New Biol. 243: 246-247, 1973a.

Donta, S.T., Moon, H.W. and Whipp, S.C.: Detection of heat-labile Escherichia coli enterotoxin with the use of adrenal cells in tissue culture. Science 183: 334-336, 1973b.

Duguid, J.P., Smith, I.W., Dempster, G. and Edmunds, P.N.: Non-flagellar filamentous appendages ('fimbriae') and haemagglutinating activity in Bacterium coli. J.Path.Bacteriol. 70: 335-348, 1955.

Duguid, J.P.: Fimbriae and adhesive properties in Klebsiella strains. J.Gen.Microbiol. 21: 271-286, 1959.

Edwards, P.R. and Ewing, W.H.: Identification of Enterobacteriaceae. Burgess Publishing Co., Minneapolis, 1972.

Evans, D.G., Evans, D.J. and Pierce, N.F.: Differences in the response of rabbit small intestine to heat-labile and heat-stable enterotoxins of Escherichia coli. Infect.Immun. 7: 873-880, 1973.

Gianella, R.A.: Suckling mouse model for detection of heat-stable Escherichia coli enterotoxin: characteristics of the model. Infect.Immun. 14: 95-99, 1976.

Guerrant, R.L., Brunton, L.L., Schnaitman, T.C., Rebhun, L.I. and Gilman, A.G.: Cyclic adenosine monophosphate and alteration of Chinese hamster ovary cell morphology: a rapid sensitive in vitro assay for the enterotoxins of Vibrio cholerae and Escherichia coli. Infect.Immun. 10: 320-327, 1974.

Guinée, P.A.M., Jansen, W.H. and Agterberg, C.M.: Detection of the K99 antigen by means of agglutination and immunoelectrophoresis in Escherichia coli isolates from calves and its correlation with enterotoxigenicity. Infect.Immun. 13: 1369-1377, 1976.

Guinée, P.A.M., Agterberg, C.M., Jansen, W.H. and Frik, J.F.: Serological identification of pig enterotoxigenic Escherichia coli strains not belonging to the classical serotypes. Infect.Immun. 15: 549-555, 1977a.

140

Guinée, P.A.M., Veldkamp, J. and Jansen, W.H.: Improved Minca medium for the detection of K99 antigen in calf enterotoxigenic strains of Escherichia coli. Infect.Immun. 15: 676-678, 1977b.

Guinée, P.A.M. and Jansen, W.H.: Behavior of Escherichia coli K antigens K88ab, K88ac and K88ad in immunoelectrophoresis, double diffusion and hemagglutination. Infect.Immun. 23: 700-705, 1979a.

Guinée, P.A.M. and Jansen, W.H.: Detection of enterotoxigenicity and attachment factors in Escherichia coli strains of human, porcine and bovine origin; a comparative study. Zbl.Bakt.Hyg., I.Abt.Orig.A 243: 245-257, 1979b.

Gyles, C.L.: Limitations of the infant mouse test for Escherichia coli heat-stable enterotoxin. Can.J.comp.Med. 43: 371-379, 1979.

Isaacson, R.E., Nagy, B. and Moon, H.W.: Colonization of porcine small intestine by Escherichia coli: colonization and adhesion factors of pig enteropathogens that lack K88. J.Infect.Dis. 135: 531-539, 1977.

Isaacson, R.E.: Factors affecting expression of the Escherichia coli pilus K99. Infect.Immun. 28: 190-194, 1980.

Jones, G.W.: The adhesive properties of K88 antigen of strains of Escherichia coli pathogenic to neonatal pigs. Ph.D.Thesis University of Reading, England.

Jones, G.W. and Rutter, J.M.: The association of K88 antigen with haemagglutinating activity in porcine strains of E.coli. J.Gen.Microbiol. 84: 135-144, 1974.

Kantor, H.S., Tao, P. and Wisdom, C.: Action of Escherichia coli enterotoxin: Adenylate cyclase behaviour of intestinal epithelial cells in culture. Infect.Immun. 9: 1003-1010, 1974.

Kimberg, D.V., Field, M., Johnson, J., Henderson, A. and Gershon, E.: Stimulation of intestinal mucosal adenyl cyclase by cholera enterotoxin and prostaglandins. J.clin.Invest. 50: 1218-1230, 1971.

Konowalchuk, J., Speirs, J.I. and Stavric, S.: Vero response to a cytotoxin of Escherichia coli. Infect.Immun. 18: 775-779, 1977.

Lathe, R., Hirth, P. DeWilde, M., Harford, N. and Lecocq, J.-P.: Cell-free synthesis of enterotoxin of E.coli from a cloned gene. Nature 284: 473-474, 1980.

Mooi, F.R. and De Graaf, F.K.: Isolation and characterization of K88 antigens. FEMS Microbiol. Lett. 5: 17-20, 1979.

Moon, H.W.: Pathogenesis of enteric diseases cause by Escherichia coli. Advanc.Vet.Sci.Comp.Med. 18: 179-211, 1974.

Moon, H.W. and Whipp, S.C.: Development of resistance with age by swine intestine to effects of enteropathogenic Escherichia coli. J.Infect. Dis. 122: 220-223, 1970.

Moon, H.W., Kohler, E.M., Scheider, R.A. and Whipp, S.C.: Prevalence of pilus antigens, enterotoxin types and enteropathogenicity among K88-negative enterotoxigenic Escherichia coli from neonatal pigs. Infect. Immun. 27: 222-230, 1980.

Moon, H.W., Nagy, B., Isaacson, R.E. and Ørskov, I.: Occurrence of K99 antigen on Escherichia coli isolated from pigs and colonization of pig ileum by K99$^+$ enterotoxigenic E.coli from calves and pigs. Infect. Immun. 15: 614-620, 1977.

Myers, L.L. and Guinée, P.A.M.: Occurrence and characteristics of enterotoxigenic Escherichia coli isolated·from calves with diarrhoea. Infect. Immun. 13: 1117-1119, 1976.

Nagy, B., Moon, H.W. and Isaacson, R.E.: Colonization of porcine small intestine by Escherichia coli: ileal colonization and adhesion by pig enteropathogens that lack K88 antigen and by some acapsular mutants.

Infect.Immun. 13: 1214-1220, 1976.

Old, D.C., Corneil, I., Gibson, L.F., Thomson, A.D. and Duguid, J.P.: Fimbriation, pellicle formation and the amount of growth of salmonellas in broth. J.Gen.Microbiol. 51: 1-16, 1968.

Olssen, E. and Söderlind, O.: Comparison of different assays for definition of heat-stable enterotoxigenicity of Escherichia coli porcine strains. J.Clin.Microbiol. 11: 6-15, 1980.

Ørskov, I., Ørskov, F., Sojka, W.J. and Leach, J.N.: Simultaneous occurrence of E.coli B and L antigens in strains from diseased swine. Influence of cultivation temperature on two new E.coli K antigens K87 and K88. Acta path.microbiol.Scand. 53: 404-422, 1961.

Ørskov, I., Ørskov, F., Sojka, W.J. and Wittig, W.: K antigens K88ab(L) and K88ac(L) in Escherichia coli. Acta path.microbiol.Scand. 62: 439-447, 1964.

Ørskov, I. and Ørskov, F.: Episome carried surface antigen K88 of E.coli. I. Transmission of the determinant of the K88 antigen and the influence on the transfer of chromosomal markers. J.Bacteriol. 91: 69-75, 1966.

Ørskov, I., Ørskov, F., Williams-Smith, H. and Sojka, W.J.: The establishment of K99, a thermolabile, transmissible Escherichia coli K antigen, previously called 'Kco', possessed by calf and lamb enteropathogenic strains. Acta path.microbiol.Scand. 83: 31-36, 1975.

Ørskov, I., Ørskov, F., Jann, B. and Jann, K.: Serology, chemistry and genetics of O and K antigens of Escherichia coli. Bact.Rev. 41: 667-710, 1977.

Runnels, P.L., Moon, H.W. and Schneider, R.A.: Development of resistance with host age to adhesion of K99$^+$ Escherichia coli to isolated intestinal epithelial cells. Infect.Immun. 28: 298-300, 1980.

Sack, D.A., Huda, S., Neogi, P.K.B., Dahniel, R.R. and Spira, W.M.: Microtiter ganglioside enzyme linked immunosorbent assay for Vibrio and Escherichia coli heat-labile enterotoxins and antitoxin. J.Clin. Microbiol. 11: 35-40, 1980.

Sellwood, R., Gibbons, R.A., Jones, G.W. and Rutter, J.M.: Adhesion of enteropathogenic Escherichia coli to pig intestinal brush-borders: the existence of two pig phenotypes. J.Med.Microbiol. 8: 405-411, 1975.

Sellwood, R. and Lees, D.: Adhesion of Escherichia coli pathogenic to pigs, calves and lambs to intestinal epithelial cell brush-borders. E.E.C. Workshop, Lelystad, The Netherlands, 1980.

Smith, H.W. and Halls, S.: Studies on Escherichia coli enterotoxin. J.Path.Bacteriol. 93: 531-543, 1967.

Smith, H.W. and Halls, S.: The transmissible nature of the genetic factor in Escherichia coli that controls enterotoxin production. J.Gen. Microbiol. 52: 319-334, 1968.

Smith, H.W. and Gyles, C.L.: The relationship between two apparently different enterotoxins produced by enteropathogenic strains of Escherichia coli of porcine origin. J.Med.Microbiol. 3: 387-401, 1970a.

Smith, H.W. and Gyles, C.L.: The effect of cell-free fluids prepared from culture of human and animal enteropathogenic strains of Escherichia coli on ligated intestinal segments of rabbits and pigs. J.Med.Microbiol. 3: 403-409, 1970b.

Smith, H.W. and Linggood, M.A.: Further observations on Escherichia coli enterotoxins with particular regard to those produced by atypical piglet strains and by calf and lamb strains: the transmissible nature of these enterotoxins and of a K antigen possessed by calf and lamb strains. J.Med.Microbiol. 5: 243-250, 1972.

Smith, H.W. and Huggins, M.B.: The influence of plasmid-determined and other characteristics of enteropathogenic Escherichia coli on their ability to proliferate in the alimentary tracts of piglets, calves and lambs. J.Med.Microbiol. 11: 471-492, 1978.

Söderlind, O.: Studies on Escherichia coli in pigs. IV. Reactions of Escherichia coli strains in the ligated intestine test. Zbl.Vet.Med.B. 20: 558-571, 1973.

Söderlind, O. and Möllby, R.: Enterotoxins, O-groups and K88 antigen in Escherichia coli from neonatal piglets with and without diarrhea. Infect.Immun. 24: 611-616, 1979.

Sojka, W.J.: Escherichia coli in domestic animals and poultry. Review series no. 7 of the Commonwealth Bureau of Animal Health. The eastern press Ltd. 1965.

Speirs, J.I., Stavric, S. and Konowalchuk, J.: Assay of Escherichia coli heat-labile enterotoxin with vero cells. Infect.Immun. 16: 617-622, 1977.

Wadström, T., Aust-Kettis, A., Habte, D., Holmgren, J., Meeuwisse, G., Möllby, R. and Söderlind, O.: Enterotoxin-producing bacteria and parasites in stools of Ethiopian children with diarrhoeal disease. Arch.Dis.Childh. 51: 865-870, 1976.

Wilcock, J.: Experimental Klebsiella and Salmonella infection in neonatal swine. Canad.J.Comp.Med. 43: 700-706, 1979.

Manual 1.

Preparation of cultures, LT and ST for in vivo or in vitro assays.

Laboratory manual of the National Institute of Public Health, Laboratory
for Bacteriology, Bilthoven, The Netherlands.

The medium recommended for LT as well as ST production is that described
by Evans et al.

Casamino acids (Difco)	20	g
Yeast extract (Difco)	6	g
NaCl (p.a.)	2.5	g
KH_2PO_4 (p.a.)	8.71	g
Trace salts solution	1	ml (see manual 5)

Adjust pH to 8.5 with 0.1 NaOH.

Distilled water ad 1000 ml.

Autoclave at 121°C for 20 minutes.

Add 2.5 ml of sterile 20% glucose solution.

The strains under test are inoculated into 10 ml of medium in 60 or 100 ml
screw-capped bottles and incubated in a shaking waterbath (250 rpm) for
24 hrs. at 37°C. 100 µl of culture is transferred into 10 ml of fresh
medium and similarly incubated. Such cultures can be used in the Ligated
Gut Test. For preparation of cell-free LT and ST preparations, bacterial
cells are removed by centrifugation at 20.000 x g for 30 min. and poly-
myxin B sulphate is added to give a final concentration of 50 µg/ml.
ST toxin preparations to be used in the suckling mous test are stained
by adding two drops of 0.5% of Evans blue solution per ml supernatant.

Reference

Evans, D.G., Evans, D.J.jr. and Gorbach, S.L.: Identification of entero-
    toxigenic Escherichia coli and serum antitoxin activity by the vascu-
    lar permeability factor assay. Infect.Immun. 8: 731-735, 1973.

Manual 2.

Assay of ST in the suckling mouse test.

Laboratory manual of the National Institute of Public Health, Laboratory for Bacteriology, Bilthoven, The Netherlands.

The preparation of ST has been described in manual 1.

Infant mice at least 2 days old and not older than 4-5 days which have a well-filled and hence clearly visible stomach are selected from several litters. When selected as early in the morning as conveniently possible, sufficient mice will be found to be suitable. Other mice will become suitable later when left to suckle the mother. During the test, the mice should be left at about 30°C. The mice are injected intragastrically with 0.1 ml of Evans blue-stained ST preparation. Animals with no dye in the intestine or with dye within the peritoneal cavity at autopsy should be discarded, because the have not been injected properly.

Each strain is tested in 3-4 mice. The mice are kept at 30°C and killed after 3-4 hours by decapitation. The entire intestine (not including the stomach) is removed and inspected. The intestines of the 3-4 mice per test are pooled and weighed and the ratio of gut weight to the combined weight of the remaining carcasses is calculated. A ratio of ≤ 0.08 indicates a negative result, a ratio of ≥ 0.09 indicates a positive result. The following weighing procedure provides an extra control: 3-4 mice are weighed before sacrifice; after sacrifice the pooled intestines and the pooled carcasses (including heads and stomachs) are weighed separately. If the sum of the carcasses and intestines is less than 95% of the total body weight before sacrifice, the test should be discarded, because too much relevant material has been lost during sacrificing manipulations.

References

Dean, A., Ching, Y.C., Williams, R.G. and Harden, L.B.: Test for Escherichia coli enterotoxin using infant mice: application in a study of
diarrhea in children in Honolulu. J.Infect.Dis. 125: 407-411, 1972.

Giannella, R.A.: Suckling mouse-model for detection of heat-stable
Escherichia coli enterotoxin: characteristics of the model. Infect.
Immun. 14: 95-99, 1976.

Manual 3.

The ligated gut test (LGT) in pigs.

Laboratory manual of the Veterinary Faculty, University of Utrecht,
Utrecht, The Netherlands.

The LGT is a test to assess E.coli strains for the production of entero-
toxin (both LT and ST). Suspensions of living bacteria (cultures) as well
as cell-free preparations can be used as test material.
The pig is starved for 24 hrs. Free access to water is allowed.
Prior to full anaesthesia the pig is treated with azaperone (Stresnil,
Janssen Pharmaceutica) and methomidate (Hypnodil, Janssen Pharmaceutica)
and placed in a quiet, dark room.
About 15.minutes after the pre-anaesthetic treatment full anaesthesia is
achieved with laughing-gas and halothane.
The abdomen is opened on the right side of the pig by a dorso-ventral in-
cision of about 10 cm, just behind the last rib, while the animal lies on
its left side.
Starting about 2 m from the pylorus, segments of the small intesting alternately about 10-15 cm long and 5-10 cm long are ligated with string
ligatures.
The test materials are injected into the 10-15 cm long segments, while
the intermediate, 5-19 cm long segments serve as untreated controls.
The abdomen is closed with nylon sutures and the animal is allowed to re-
cover from anaesthesia. The analgeticum Tomanol (Byk Gulden) may be used
as a pain-killer.
The pig is killed 16-24 hrs. later by the intravenous administration of
an overdose of sodium pentobarbital (Triotal, Gist-Brocades). Usually 16
hrs. will be sufficient.
The abdomen is opened and the small intestine carefully removed and un-
ravelled.
The presence or absence of dilatation is recorded, as well as the length
of the dilated segments.
The fluid contents of each dilated segment is collected and the weight of
the contents in grams or the amount of the contents in milliliters is
determined.
Usually a reaction is recorded as positive if the LGT index (amount of

fluid in milliliters or grams/length of the segment in cm) $\geq$ 1. The strain inoculated has to be reisolated from the segment in question.

The anterior part of the small intestine is more susceptible to dilatation than the posterior part, therefore the last 3 m should not be used. About 40 tests may be done in one animal.

It is recommended to apply positive and negative controls every 10 segments. A reaction in a particular segment may then be considered to be reliable when the distal and proximal positive and negative controls give the proper reactions.

Addendum

If one wishes to make intra vitam observations, e.g. on the time-related emergence of fluid accumulation, full anaesthesia should be prolonged until final autopsy. Heartrate and blood pressure etc. should then be monitored. For this purpose, the arteria carotis and the vena maxillaris externa are prepared free on the right side. The arteria carotis is used for monitoring the heartrate, and the diastolic and systolic pressure and for taking bloodsamples to determine the pCO_2, pO_2 and the base excess. Plasma or Ringer's solution may be infused into the vena maxillaris externa.

Manual 4.

Assay of LT in the Vero cell test.

Laboratory manual of the National Institute of Public Health, Laboratory for Bacteriology, Bilthoven, The Netherlands.

LT is prepared as described in manual 1.

Monolayers are grown in a 25 well tissue culture plate (Sterilin 306V) by inoculation of each well with 1 ml containing 1×10^5 Vero cells in medium 199 plus Earle salts and 5% neonatal calf serum (Flow) containing 12.5 μg/ml kanamycin. The 25 well plate is incubated for 2-3 days at $37^{\circ}C$ in a humidified atmosphere of 5% CO_2 in air, resulting in confluent monolayers. Thirty minutes prior to the experiment, the culture medium is replaced by the same medium without calf serum, but containing 0.05 mM methyl-isobu-tyl-xanthine (Aldrich-Europe, Belgium) as phosphordiesterase inhibitor. After 30 minutes, 25 μl of each of the LT preparations to be tested is added to a well. The plate is read after 24 hrs. incubation under an inverted microscope with phase contrast attachment. Proper controls such as LT plus (positive control), LT minus and heated (15' $100^{\circ}C$) LT plus preparations (negative control) as well as uninoculated wells should be included. LT causes rounding of the Vero cells.

References

Konowalchuk, J., Speirs, J.I. and Stavric, S.: Vero response to a cyto-toxin of Escherichia coli. Infect.Immun. 18: 775-779, 1977.
Speirs, J.I., Stavric, S. and Konowalchuk, J.: Assay of Escherichia coli heat-labile enterotoxin with vero cells. Infect.Immun. 16: 617-622, 1977.

Manual 5.

Production of the adhesins K88, K99 and P987.

Laboratory manual of the National Institute of Public Health, Laboratory
for Bacteriology, Bilthoven, The Netherlands.

1. K88.

All three serological varieties (K88ab, K88ac and K88ad) of the K88
adhesin are equally well produced on common nutrient media such as 5%
sheep blood agar as well as on Minca-IsoVitalex agar (see Section 2)
at $37^\circ C$.

2. K99.

In terms of detectibility by means of slide agglutination, the K99
adhesin is sufficiently produced only when cultured on Minca-IsoVitalex
medium. Minca Is-medium is composed as follows:

KH_2PO_4 (p.a.)	1.36	g
$Na_2HPO_4 \cdot 2H_2O$ (p.a.)	10.1	g
casamino-acids (Difco)	1	g
Trace salts solution	1	g
agar (Difco)	12	g
aqua dest	1000	ml
IsoVitalex (BBL)	1	ampoule
pH 7.5		

The trace salts solution contains per 1000 ml:

$MgSO_4 \cdot 7H_2O$ (p.a.)	10	g
$MnCl_2 \cdot 4H_2O$ (p.a.)	1	g
$FeCl_3 \cdot 6H_2O$ (p.a.)	0.135	g
$CaCl_2 \cdot 2H_2O$ (p.a.)	0.4	g
Sterilize at $100^\circ C$.		

A practical procedure for the preparation of 1000 ml of Minca-Is medium
is to compose it from prefabricated and presterilized stocks:

Stock 1. Trace salts solution (see above).

Stock 2.	KH_2PO_4	2.72 g
	$Na_2HPO_4 \cdot 2H_2O$	20.2 g

Dissolve in 1000 ml aqua dest and sterilize at 100°C.

Stock 3. Casamino acids 5 g in 100 ml.

Sterilize at 121°C for 20 min.

Stock 4. Agar 26 g in 1000 ml.

Sterilize at 121°C for 20 min.

Mix: Stock 1   1 ml

Stock 2   500 ml prewarmed to 50°C

Stock 3   20 ml

Stock 4   460 ml prewarmed to 50°C

Add: one ampoule of lyophilized IsoVitalex in 10 ml of its glucose-containing solvent (Polyvitex, Merieux France has equal activity as IsoVitalex).

Mix and pour plates and/or slopes.

3. P987.

The P987 adhesin can be detected by slide agglutination from 5% sheep blood agar plates inoculated from faeces or intestinal contents. However, usually not more than 10% of the colonies carry the P987 adhesin. Moreover, on further subculturing the P987 adhesin is usually no longer expressed. However, if Slanetz medium (manual 8) is used, P987 colonies can easily be subcultured and the proportion of piliated colonies increased to at least 99%. An alternative method to enrich for P987[+] bacteria in laboratory cultures is inoculation into 10 ml of nutrient broth enriched with 10% horse serum in 18x200 mm tubes. After incubation at 37°C without shaking for about one week P987[+] strains will show either a pellicle or a loose deposit on the bottom of the tube. If so, preferentially the pellicle is subcultured on nutrient agar with 5% sheep blood. The resulting growth can then be tested for the presence of the P987 antigen by means of the slide agglutination. Cultures grown at 18°C should be negative in the slide agglutination.

References

Guinée, P.A.M., Veldkamp, J. and Jansen, W.H.: Improved Minca medium for the detection of K99 antigen in calf enterotoxigenic strains of Escherichia coli. Infect.Immun. 15: 676-678, 1977b.

Isaacson, R.E., Nagy, B. and Moon, H.W.: Colonization of porcine small intestine by Escherichia coli: colonization and adhesion factors of pig enteropathogens that lack K88. J.Infect.Dis. 135: 531-539, 1977.

Manual 6.

A. Preparation of E.coli O, K and H antisera; a general outline.
B. Principles of serotyping of E.coli.
C. Preparation of antisera for the detection of bovine and porcine entero-
   pathogenic E.coli strains.

Laboratory manual of the National Institute of Public Health, Laboratory
for Bacteriology, Bilthoven, The Netherlands.

A. Preparation of E.coli O, K and H antisera; a general outline (see
   references 1 and 8).

   A.1. O antisera

   A smooth colony is inoculated into nutrient broth and incubated
   for 6-8 hrs. at 37°C and then heated at 100°C for 2½ hrs. This
   procedure inactivates all other antigens except the O antigen.
   Cultures possessing a K antigen of the A variety are not used for
   O antiserum production. Only suspensions that are homogeneous and
   not autoagglutinable upon heating, are selected for inoculation
   into rabbits. Two rabbits should be injected with each antigen in
   the marginal ear vein. Doses of 0.5 ml, 1 ml, 2 ml and 3-4 ml respectively are given at 4-5 days intervals. The animals are proof-
   bled or exsanguinated 6-8 days after the last injection. The sera
   are separated and preserved by addition of a suitable preservative
   (NaN₃ 0.1%; merthiolate 0.001%). Antigens to be used for testing O
   antisera are prepared as described above. Agglutination tests
   should be incubated in a waterbath at about 50°C for 16-18 hrs.
   Titers obtainable with O antisera vary widely but may reach
   1:10,000 in tube agglutination tests. Instead of tubes, disposable
   trays are being used for this purpose (reference 2). O antisera
   should be checked for specificity by testing them against all
   known O antigens (O1-O163). Aspecific reactions may be removed by
   absorption with heterologous antigen(s) (see reference 1).

   A.2. K antisera (with the exception of K88, K99 and P987; see part C
              of this manual)
   Unheated cells either living of formalin-killed have to be used
   for immunization in order not to inactivate the K antigen.

This means that antibodies will also be formed against all other antigenic determinants of the immunizing strain including the O antigen and H antigen, if the strain is motile. Therefore, either non-motile strains should be used or methods employed, which decrease the immunogenicity of the H antigen (see reference 1). Even then, such K antisera may yield up to 10 precipitation lines in addition to the K line when tested in immunoelectrophoresis against ultrasonicates of the homologous strain. K^+ colonies are selected for vaccine production and transferred to agar slants. The first injection is given with cells killed with 0.5% formalin for 24 hrs., the second injection with cells treated for 2 hrs. with 0.5% formalin and the following injections with living cells. The immunization scheme is similar to that described for O antisera. Broth cultures obtained from K^+ colonies, incubated 6-8 hrs. at 37°C and then formalinised are used as antigens and added to serial dilutions of antisera ranging from 1:20 to 1:2500. The tests are incubated at 37°C for 2 hrs. followed by overnight incubation at 4°C. A typical K agglutination is characterized by the formation of a disc or pellicle at the bottom of the tube. Titers are recorded as the highest dilution giving good disc formation. Titers of 1:60 to 1:640 may be obtained. Such antisera may be used in dilutions of 1:5 to 1:20 for slide agglutination tests. K antisera should be checked for homologous O and H antibodies. High titers of H antibodies may cause aspecific reactions. Also antigenic relationships between K antigens and antisera have been described, due to polysaccharide K antigens proper or due to other, non-specified, surface antigens. The preparation of specific K antisera is therefore a tedious job.

A.3. H antisera

H antigens for production and control of antisera are prepared from highly motile cultures which have been selected by passage through U-tubes with semi-solid nutrient medium (0.1%-0.4% agar). After about 5 passages, the culture is grown in nutrient broth at 37°C for 15-18 hrs. and then formalinized (0.5%). The immunization scheme is similar to that described for O antisera. Tests for H agglutination are incubated in a waterbath at 50°C and read after

1 hour. The agglutinate is very loose. Titers of 1:10,000 are
usually obtained. The height of the H antigen titer and the short
incubation time prevent aspecific reactions due to 0, K or other
antigens.

B. Principles of serotyping of E.coli.

  B.1. Complete serotyping

    B.1.1. A boiled broth culture of the strain to be typed is tested
against all O antisera in tube agglutination tests. This is
usually done in steps. The O antisera in an appropriate
dilution have been divided into about 20 pools. The heated
broth culture is tested against the pools. In the second
step the broth culture is tested against the individual
O antisera in appropriated dilution contained in the
pool(s) in which the broth culture gave a positive reaction.
Finally, the broth culture is tested against serial dilutions of the O antiserum or antisera showing agglutination
in the second step. Thus, the O antigen group is established. Since this procedure is still quite laborious, successful attempts to mechanize the procedure have been made (2).

    B.1.2. The growth of a fresh agar slant is used for the K antigen
determination. The slant is agglutinated by slide agglutination against an appropriate dilution of its homologous O
antiserum. Positive agglutination indicates the absence of
a K antigen. If negative, the slant is tested against the
K antisera known to be associated with that O group. If
positive, the K antigen is provisionally established. If
negative, the result is recorded as K? indicating a surface
structure causing O inagglutinability. It has been felt
that this procedure is not watertight in several respects.

      a. The positive agglutination test should be confirmed by
immuno- or counter-immunoelectrophoresis tests (CIE)
using a 100°C extract of a suspension of the strain under test to confirm the presence of a polysaccharide K
antigen (7).

      b. Testing of a strain with a particular O antigen against

K antisera "known to be associated" with that O group
has limited value, because the relation between O and
K antigen in E.coli strains has been established empiri-
cally rather than systematically. Attempts to test each
E.coli strain against all K antisera using a mechanised
technique (2) met with many atypical reactions which
have to be confirmed in CIE.

B.1.3. For H antigen determination, the culture under test has to
be checked for motility in U tubes and if motile, passed
through U tubes about 3-5 times. After the last passage,
a nutrient broth is inoculated and treated as described for
H antiserum production. The suspension is tested against
(pools of) the H antisera and titrated as described for the
O antigen determination.

B.2. Partial serotyping

This method is often used in order to detect whether a particular
isolate belongs to a pathogenic E.coli type, making use of the
partially established correlation between pathogenicity and serotype. In contrast to complete serotyping, partial serotyping may
also be successfully carried out in less specialised laboratories.
For this purpose, one preferably employs OK antisera (separate or
in pools) and non-heated agar cultures in the slide agglutination
test. The diagnosis of enteropathogenic E.coli types associated
with human infantile diarrhoea is set out here as an example. The
following serotypes are often associated with infantile diarrhoea
(incomplete list!): O26:(K60)
                     O55:(K59)
                     O125:(K70)
                     O128:(K67)
A suspected culture in the living state is tested by slide agglutination in a pool containing all four OK antisera. If positive,
the culture is tested in the separate OK antisera. If the strain
is agglutinated by one antiserum only and not by the other sera,
the OK antigen has been determined with a high probability, ex-
cluding autoagglutinability. However, because of the natural

aspecificity of OK antisera, a heated broth culture of the strain
under test should be tested in tube dilution test against pure O
antiserum.

C. Preparation of antisera for the detection of bovine and porcine enteropathogenic E.coli strains.

    C.1. The general procedures outlined in Section A of this manual are
also valid for the production of antisera mentioned in the title
except K88, K99 and P987 antisera. For the production of OK antisera meant for serotyping of the classical porcine serotypes and
bovine strains, strains devoid of the K88 and K99 antigen should
be used. Such strains are often found as natural isolates and are
also available as reference strains. If not available, strains for
antiserum production should be cultured at $20^\circ C$ to prevent formation of K88 or K99 antigen. Since the detection of the K88, K99
and P987 antigen has particular diagnostic significance, special
attention is given to the production of specific antisera against
these adhesins.

    C.2. **Production of K88 antisera**

It should be borne in mind that K88 occurs in three varieties
K88ab, K88ac, K88ad.

        C.2.1. The procedure for production of OK antisera as outlined in
Section A of this manual can also be employed for the production of K88 antisera. Vaccines are obtained from K88-
rich, wild-type or reference strains. Proof-bleedings are
tested for their K88 antibody content by slide agglutination against homologous and heterologous (other serotypes
with K88 antigen) strains. The antiserum should be absorbed
with the homologous culture grown at $20^\circ C$ to render it sufficiently specific. Specificity of the absorbed antiserum
should be controlled by slide agglutination against homologous and heterologous cultures ($K88^+$ and $K88^-$) grown at
$37^\circ C$ and $20^\circ C$ or by means of immunodiffusion tests (5).
Specific K88ab, K88ac and K88ad antisera should be appropriately pooled in order to ensure sufficiently strong

reactions with all three K88 varieties. This method of
rendering K88 antisera specific is rather laborious. The
growth of one 15 cm diameter nutrient agar plate incubated
at 20°C for 48 hrs. is required for proper absorption of
1 ml of undiluted antiserum.

C.2.2. The use of K88^{+} E.coli K12 transconjugants for immunization
offers the advantage that generally less heterologous antibodies are formed and that the antisera may be absorbed
with E.coli K12 grown at 37°C. The remaining procedures
are identical to those under 2.1.

C.2.3. Several attempts have been made to purify the K88 antigen
(9). Attempts to prepare specific K88 antisera were successful for K88ab and K88ad, but failed for K88ac ("Preparation of E.coli K88 antisera by means of purified K88ab
and K88ad antigens"; Guinée, Mooi and Jansen, accepted for
publication, Zbl.Bakt.).
Monospecific K88b, K88c and K88d antisera may be obtained
by similar absorptions.

C.3. Production of K99 antiserum

Similar procedures as described for K88 antiserum may be used for
K99 antiserum production. The strain for production should be
grown on Minca Is-medium at 37°C. The strain for absorption of the
crude antiserum may be grown on common nutrient medium at 20°C.
However, the laborious absorption of crude antisera can be avoided
by using K99 antigen purified by means of preparative electrophoresis (3). Generally, antisera for slide agglutination tests are
appropriately diluted with 0.5% phenol in 0.5% NaCl solution. K99
antiserum was found to yield clearer agglutination reactions when
diluted with buffered NaCl solution (1M NaCl in 0.022 M Sörensen
phosphate buffer, pH 7.3, merthiolate 0.001%). A control reaction
in normal rabbit antiserum similarly diluted as the K99 antiserum
is required to exclude autoagglutinability.

C.4. Production of P987 antiserum

Production of P987 pili by P987$^+$ strains can be promoted by the pellicle-producing procedure described in manual 5. The following technique enabled us to prepare a satisfactorily strong and specific P987 antiserum. Pellicles of a P987$^+$ strain obtained in static horseserum enriched broth cultures were thoroughly suspended in 0.066 M Sörensen phosphate buffer, pH 7.3 to give a concentration of 1 x 10^9 (E 600 nm = 1.0). Rabbits were injected intravenously with increasing volumes (0.5 - 4 ml) of formalin-killed or living cells at 4-5 days intervals, as described for K antiserum production. Proof bleedings were evaluated by means of immunodiffusion (ID) and immunoelectrophoresis (IE) tests in Noble agar gel using ultrasonicates of P$^+$ cells grown at 37°C (US 37) and 18°C (US 18) (6). After 4-6 injections, the proof bleedings showed an extra precipitation line against homologous US 37 when compared with US 18. The rabbits were bled and the antisera absorbed with an equal volume of US 18. All antibodies against US 18 were thus removed and the remaining, single precipitation line against US 37 was considered to represent P987 antibody. This antiserum could be used in the slide agglutination test in a dilution of 1:5. For details of preparation of ultrasonicates, ID and IE, the reader is referred to the original literature (3, 4).

C.5. Final remarks

C.5.1. It has become standard procedure in our Laboratory to use for antiserum production only rabbits which have been selected for the absence of antibodies to E.coli by testing proof bleedings in immunodiffusion tests against US 37 of a number of strains before immunization (5).

C.5.2. To our knowledge, antisera for the detection of animal enteropathogenic strains are not commercially available. The following antisera are available at a limited level from the National Institute of Public Health, P.O.Box 1, 3720 BA Bilthoven, The Netherlands.
   1. 0138:(K81)
   2. 0139:K82

3. 0141:(K85ab)

4. 0141:(K85ac)

5. 08:K87

6. 0147:(K89)

7. 0149:(K91)

8. Specific K88 (containing K88 ac and K88ad and sufficiently reacting also with K88ab).

9. Polyvalent antiserum containing 1-7 and K88 antibodies.

10. K99 and control serum.

References

1. Edwards, P.R. and Ewing, W.H.: Identification of Enterobacteriaceae.
   Burgess Publishing Co., Minneapolis, 1972.
2. Guinée, P.A.M., Agterberg, C.M. and Jansen, W.H.: Escherichia coli O
   antigen typing by means of a mechanised microtechnique. Appl.Micro-
   biol. 24: 127-131, 1972.
3. Guinée, P.A.M., Jansen, W.H. and Agterberg, C.M.: Detection of the K99
   antigen by means of agglutination and immunoelectrophoresis in
   Escherichia coli isolates from calves and its correlation with ente--
   rotoxigenicity. Infect.Immun. 13: 1369-1377, 1976.
4. Guinée, P.A.M., Agterberg, C.M., Jansen, W.H. and Frik, J.F.: Serological identification of pig enterotoxigenic Escherichia coli strains
   not belonging to the classical serotypes. Infect.Immun. 15: 549-555,
   1977.
5. Guinée, P.A.M. and Jansen, W.H.: Behavior of Escherichia coli K antigens K88ab, K88ac and K88ad in immunoelectrophoresis, double diffusion and hemagglutination. Infect.Immun. 23: 700-705, 1979.
6. Guinée, P.A.M. and Jansen, W.H.: Detection of enterotoxigenicity and
   attachment factors in Escherichia coli strains of human, porcine and
   bovine origin; a comparative study. Zbl.Bakt.Hyg., I.Abt.Orig. A 243:
   245-257, 1979.
7. Semjen, G., Ørskov, I. and Ørskov, F.: K antigen determination of
   Escherichia coli by counter-current immunoelectrophoresis (CIE). Acta
   Path.Microbiol. scand.Sect.B.: 103-107, 1977.
8. Sojka, W.J.: Escherichia coli in domestic animals and poultry. Review
   series no. 7 of the Commonwealth Bureau of Animal Health. The Eastern
   press Ltd. 1965.
9. Stirm, S., Ørskov, I., Ørskov, F. and Mansa, B.: Episome-carried surface antigen K88 of Escherichia coli. II Isolation and chemical
   analysis. J.Bact. 93: 731-739, 1967.

158

Manual 7.

A. Bacteriological techniques recommended for the detection of enterotoxigenic E.coli strains in calves in diagnostic field-laboratories.
B. Bacteriological techniques recommended for the detection of enterotoxigenic E.coli strains in neonatal and post-weaning E.coli enterotoxin
   induced diarrhoea (and oedema-disease) in piglets.

Laboratory manual of the Central Veterinary Institute, Department for
Bacteriology, Rotterdam, The Netherlands.

A. Bacteriological techniques recommended for the detection of enterotoxigenic E.coli strains in calves in diagnostic field-laboratories.
   Until now a nearly 100% positive correlation between the K99-adhesive
   antigen and the ability to produce ST has been found in strains of
   bovine origin.
   Up to now K99 is the only known adhesive antigen in bovine enterotoxigenic E.coli strains. So routine search for enterotoxigenic E.coli
   strains in materials of bovine origin is based on the detection of the
   K99 antigen which is optimally produced on Minca-IsoVitalex medium. It
   is therefore strongly recommended to use Minca-IsoVitalex also for
   primary isolation of suspected strains from intestinal contents.
   Materials:
   1) Minca-IsoVitalex (Minca-Is): see manual 5;
   2) agglutinating anti-K99 serum (manual 6), appropriately diluted in
      0.022 M phosphate buffer, pH 7.3, containing 1 M NaCl;
   3) control serum: normal serum of the same animal species as under 2,
      devoid of E.coli antibodies and diluted in the same way and degree
      as the anti-K99 serum;
   4) selective media for E.coli e.g. McConkey.
   Practical performance:
   1) Inoculate Minca-Is plates and selective medium with a loop of faecal
      sample or intestinal contents (taken from the anterior, middle and
      posterior small intestine).
   2) Incubate the plates overnight at 37°C.
   3) Check Minca-Is plates for K99-positive E.coli by the slide aggluti-
      nation test.
   4) Slide agglutination test: a drop of K99 antiserum is brought onto a

glass slide. A loop of bacterial growth is streaked onto the slide for 2-3 seconds and mixed with the antiserum. If the culture is rubbed on the slide without antiserum for more than 5 seconds, the reaction may be significantly weaker. If the mixture remains turbid, the agglutination test is negative; it is recommended to continue as described under 8. Formation of particles visible with the naked eye indicates a positive reaction;

5) In the latter case 3-5 isolated colonies are subcultured: each colony is transfered onto 2 Minca-Is slants or plates.

6) One slant is incubated at $37^{\circ}C$, the other one at $18-20^{\circ}C$.

7) The next day agglutinate the slant cultures incubated at $37^{\circ}C$ in K99 antiserum. If no agglutination occurs, K99 is not present. If positive, handle and interprete the results as indicated in the following scheme:

Culture incubated			
at $37^{\circ}C$		at $18^{\circ}C$	
Reaction in K99 antiserum	Reaction in control serum	Reaction in K99 antiserum	Interpretation
+	−	−	K99 positive
+	+	n.d.[*]	autoagglutinable K99 not indicated.
+	−	+	aspecific reaction K99 not indicated
−	n.d.	n.d.	K99 negative

[*] n.d.: not (to be) done.

8) If only a few colonies of the primary culture are K99-positive, they possibly are not detected under 3. To detect these small numbers, 8-10 E.coli-suspected colonies from the selective medium, if possible of various morphology, are subcultured on Minca-Is plates, incubated at $37^{\circ}C$ and tested for K99 (see 4-8). K99-bearing E.coli strains of bovine origin often are OK-types with a mucoid colony morphology.

9) If there is a strong suspicion of E.coli enterotoxin-induced diarrhoea, an attempt can be made to detect K99 by a cultural passage procedure in a last resort. If negative, subcultures should be sent to a specialised laboratory for enterotoxin assays.

B. Bacteriological techniques recommended for the detection of enterotoxigenic E.coli strains in neonatal and post-weaning E.coli enterotoxin-
induced diarrhoea (and oedema-disease) in piglets.

So far 3 adhesive antigens are known in enterotoxigenic E.coli strains
of porcine origin, i.e. K88, K99 and P987.

It should be stressed that some so-called typical or classical strains,
devoid of K88, may be encountered in cases of E.coli enterotoxin-induced diarrhoea. The majority of such strains produce one or more enterotoxins. In such cases, the correlation between OK type and production
of enterotoxin(s) can be used for the diagnosis. However, one has to
bear in mind, that enterotoxigenic E.coli strains without (known or
unknown) adhesins need not to be enteropathogenic.

So routine search for enterotoxigenic E.coli strains in samples of
porcine origin cannot be based on the detection of the K88, K99 and
P987 antigens in isolated E.coli strains only.

Materials:
1) 5% sheep blood agar plates
2) Minca-Is plates
3) a set[*] of agglutinating E.coli antisera consisting of:
   a. appropriately diluted specific (manual 5)
      OK antisera: O8:K87
                   O138:(K81)
                   O141:(K85ab)
                   O141:(K85ac)
                   O147:(K89)
                   O149:(K91)
                   O139:K82[**]
   b. appropriately diluted anti K88 serum (manual 5)
   c. polyvalent serum (Pol): directed against all OK types under a.
      + K88
   d. anti K99 serum + control serum (see under calves)
   e. anti P987 serum + control serum

---

[*] in The Netherlands produced by the National Institute of Public
    Health (see manual 6).
[**] strains with OK type O139:K82 are usually non-enterotoxigenic.
    However, ST-producing strains have been described recently. Of
    course these strains are also encountered in oedema-disease.

Practical performance:

1) Inoculate blood agar plates and Minca-Is plates with a loop of faecal sample or intestinal contents (taken from the anterior, middle and posterior small intestine).

2) Incubate the plates overnight at 37°C.

3) Check blood agar plates (and/or Minca-Is plates) for the "classical OK types" by slide agglutination in polyvalent antiserum (Pol). These strains often are β-haemolytic, but not always.

4) If an agglutination occurs, proceed with step 5. If not, proceed with step 9.

5) Agglutinate in anti K88 serum, if positive proceed with step 6; if negative proceed with step 8;

6) Each of 3-5 isolated colonies are transferred onto 2 Minca-Is slants; subsequently one slant is incubated at 37°C overnight, the other at 18-20°C.

7) If one or more of these cultures, incubated at 37°C, agglutinate(s) in anti K88 serum the following control reaction should be done: the culture grown at 18°C should not agglutinate in K88 antiserum.
This combination of reactions is indicative for the presence of K88 antigen. Proceed with step 8.

8) It is worthwhile to establish the OK type of the strain under test, particularly so when the strain is negative in anti K88 serum. OK typing of K88$^-$(Pol$^+$) cultures can be done using the primary isolation plates, but working with subcultures obtained from isolated colonies is to be preferred.
For OK typing of K88$^+$ cultures, cultures grown at 20°C are preferred, because the K88 antigen may mask the OK antigen, when grown at 37°C.

9) In case of a negative reaction in Pol, the Minca-Is plate is tested for K99$^+$ colonies as described under "calves".

10) If the strain does not react in Pol and is K99-negative, check for P987, for which the reader is referred to manual 5.

If the strains do not react in Pol, K99 or P987 and there is a strong suspicion of E.coli enterotoxin-induced diarrhoea an attempt can be made to detect K88, K99, P987 by a cultural passage procedure and pellicle formation procedure as described in the chapter on "Escherichia coli associated with neonatal diarrhoea in piglets and claves". If negative, subcultures should be sent to a specialised laboratory for enterotoxin assays.

ADHESION OF ESCHERICHIA COLI PATHOGENIC IN PIGS, CALVES AND LAMBS TO INTESTINAL EPITHELIAL CELL BRUSH-BORDERS

R. Sellwood and D. Lees*

Agricultural Research Council

Institute for Research on Animal Diseases

Compton Nr Newbury Berks RG16 ONN

*Department of Microbiology

University of Surrey

Guildford England

ABSTRACT

A study was made of the ability of K88$^+$, K99$^+$ and P987$^+$ Escherichia coli strains to attach to intestinal brush-borders prepared from different species. The K88$^+$ strain attached well only to genetically susceptible pigs. In contrast the K99$^+$ E. coli strain attached to brush-borders of all species tested except guinea pig brush-borders. The P987$^+$ strain also attached to most species; calf brush-borders being the only ones which did not show attachment.

Studies on the attachment of K99$^+$ E. coli to brush-borders prepared from calf small intestine revealed low levels of attachment in the duodenum rising to a sharp peak of attachment in the lower jejunum and again dropping to lower levels in the ileum. There was great variation in the attachment of K99$^+$ E. coli to brush-borders prepared from young lambs and no attachment was seen to brush-borders from adult sheep.

INTRODUCTION

The adhesive ability of E. coli has been known for some time but the implications of adhesive properties with intestinal infection have only recently been recognised. The ability to adhere to a cell surface can be of major ecological importance by giving the organisms, which have this ability to adhere, an advantage over the remaining bacterial flora of the tract cell surface. Many E. coli infections of the intestinal tract in both man and animals cause diarrhoea and often death in the young animal, and many of these E. coli strains have the ability to adhere (Arbuckle, 1970; Bertschinger et al., 1972; Drees & Waxler, 1970; Evans et al., 1973; Nagy et al., 1976; Smith and Linggood, 1972).

E. coli strains which have adhesive properties possess surface antigens which probably bind to the microvillus membrane of the cell. In the pig the E. coli strains most commonly isolated from the infected

neonate are those which possess the K88 antigen. Other E. coli possessing
the 987 pilus antigen are also pathogenic in pigs as well as those
possessing the K99 antigen which is more commonly associated with calf
diarrhoea.

There are two basic techniques that have been used to detect surface
antigens in vitro: (a) haemagglutination (Duguid et al., 1955; Jones &
Rutter, 1974) and (b) adhesion assays in which intestinal epithelial cells,
either as slices of intestinal tissue (Jones & Rutter, 1972) or as
isolated epithelial cells (Jones, 1972; Wilson & Hohman, 1974), are mixed
with the bacteria under investigation; and adhesion assessed either by
counting the viable organisms attached or microscopically.

Described in this paper are tests of the ability of K88[+], K99[+] and
P987[+] organisms to adhere to brush-borders prepared from the intestinal
epithelial cells of different species of animals; and the susceptibility
of the host's cells to attachment of bacteria will be discussed.

MATERIALS AND METHODS

Brush-borders were prepared (Sellwood et al., 1975) from the mucosal
cells of the jejunum or ileum of the small intestine of pigs at 16 weeks
of age. They were taken also from eight representative sites equidistant
along the small intestine from the duodenum to the ileocaecal valve of
calves at 2-3 days of age and lambs at 19 to 39 days. The whole of the
small intestine of rabbits and guinea pigs was used for the preparation
of brush-borders. Brush-borders were resuspended in 0.05M phosphate
buffered saline (PBS) pH 7.4 to a concentration of 1 x 10^6 B.B./ml for the
adhesion test or to 2.5 x 10^7/ml for the ^{3}H-labelled bacteria adhesion
assay.

Bacterial Cultures

E. coli strains were cultured according to the surface antigen being
investigated. The E. coli strain Wl (O149: K91(B), K88ac(L):H10)
producing the K88 antigen was cultured for 18 hrs at 37°C in nutrient
broth. The K99-positive strain B41 (O101:K99) was grown on tryptose
glucose yeast extract agar, TEM (Schlechts & Westphal, 1966; modified
according to Burrows et al., 1976) for 18 hrs at 37°C. The strain
possessing the 987 pilus antigen (O9:K103, P987[+]) was grown on tryptose
glucose agar (Slanetz) for 18 hrs at 37°C.

The broth cultures were centrifuged for 1000 x g for 10 min. The
solid agar cultures were harvested into PBS solution and centrifuged for
1000 x g for 10 min. The pellets were resuspended in PBS to a

concentration of 1 x 10^9 cfu/ml for use in the adhesion test.

Adhesion Test

100 µl brush-border suspension were added to 100 µl bacterial suspension in a small vial. After mixing slowly for 30 min at room temperature the suspension was viewed by phase contrast microscopy. An adhesion index was allotted to each test: - no bacteria attached/brush-border, + 1 or 2 bacteria/brush-border, ++ 3-6 bacteria/brush-border, +++ 7-12 bacteria/brush-border, ++++ 13-20 bacteria/brush-border and complete agglutination of brush-borders.

^{3}H-labelled E. coli adhesion assay

The variation in attachment of K99-positive E. coli to brush-borders prepared from different areas of small intestine in calves and sheep was studied as follows. E. coli strain B41 was cultured overnight in nutrient broth. 50 µCi ^{3}H-labelled amino acid mixture (Radiochemical Centre, Amersham, England) was added to 200 µl of culture. This bacterial suspension was used to inoculate a TEM agar plate and was incubated for 18 hrs at 37°C. The bacteria were harvested into PBS and resuspended to give a radioactive count of approximately 4 x 10^6 DPM/ml.

200 µl aliquots of formaldehyde treated brush-borders (Sellwood, 1980) were incubated with 50 µl of ^{3}H-labelled E. coli for 30 mins with gentle mixing at room temperature. The suspension was layered on to a preformed density gradient prepared by centrifugation of 7.5 ml of 45% Percoll (Pharmacia, Uppsala, Sweden) in 0.25 M sucrose for 30 mins at 56,400 x g in a 10 x 10 ml angle rotor (M.S.E. Crawley, England).

The gradient was centrifuged again for 1 hr at 16,000 x g and divided into two fractions. The upper layer contained the brush-borders with attached bacteria and the lower layer contained the excess bacteria which did not adhere. The upper layer was filtered through an 8 µm cellulose acetate filter (Millipore, Molsheim, France) and washed on the filter with 10 ml distilled water. The filter was placed in 10 ml of scintillation fluid containing 10% v/v soluene 350 and counted using an LKB Beta scintillation counter (L.K.B., Stockholm, Sweden).

RESULTS

E. coli strains possessing the surface antigens K88, K99 and 987 pilus antigen readily attached to brush-borders of certain species (Table 1). The K88$^+$ strain only adhered well to the microvillus surface of brush-borders prepared from certain specific genotypes of pig notably those being homozygous dominant (Gibbons et al., 1977) but not to homozygous

TABLE 1 - ADHESION OF <u>E. COLI</u> TO INTESTINAL BRUSH-BORDERS OF DIFFERENT
　　　　　　SPECIES

E. coli	Animal Species					
	Pig$^{(a)}$	Pig$^{(b)}$	Calf	Sheep	Rabbit	Guinea Pig
K88$^+$	++++	−	−	−	+	−
K88$^-$	−	−	−	−	−	−
K99$^+$	++++	++++	++++	+	+++	−
P987$^+$	++++	++++	−	+	++++	++++

(a) Homozygous dominant pigs　　　(b)　Homozygous recessive pigs

recessive pigs. There was some adhesion also to rabbit brush-borders but
this was minimal. The K88$^-$ mutant did not attach to brush-borders from
any species. The K99$^+$ strain adhered well to all species tested except
guinea pigs. It also adhered to both homozygous dominant and homozygous
recessive pigs. The 987 piliated strain also adhered well to most species,
the calf being the only exception.

The results of testing brush-borders prepared from sections of
intestines from sheep and lambs showed that there was great variation in
the adhesion of K99$^+$ bacteria along the length of the intestine (Table 2).
There was also no attachment to brush-borders from any section of small
intestine of the adult sheep although there was minimal attachment to the
brush-borders of the intestine of the sheep used in Table 1.

It was also evident that in any test with the K99$^+$ strain and the 987
piliated strain there was always a proportion of brush-borders which did
not have attached bacteria. This occurred in all species where there was
attachment. This phenomenon did not occur with the K88$^+$ strain with the
homozygous dominant pig in which bacteria adhered to every brush-border.

The ^{3}H-labelled K99$^+$ E. coli adhesion assay enabled the simple
adhesion test to be quantitated and showed more clearly the extent of
adherence to brush-borders prepared from different areas of small
intestine of the calf. In the calf it was found that little adhesion
occurred to the duodenum. This increased towards the posterior small
intestine but there was a sharp drop in attachment just anterior to the
ileocaecal valve. This result was typical of all the ten calves which

TABLE 2 - ADHESION OF K99+ E. COLI TO OVINE INTESTINAL BRUSH-BORDERS

Section of small intestine	Adhesion Index				
	Sheep	Lambs			
		A	B	C	D
1 (duo.)	-	++	+	-	++
2	-	+	++	-	+++
3	-	+	++	-	++
4	-	-	++	-	-
5	-	-	-	-	-
6	-	-	-	-	-
7	-	++	-	-	-
8 (il.)	-	+++	+++	+++	-

- no attachment,   + to ++++ degrees of attachment

were tested.

Fig. 1 shows the results of the quantitative adhesion assays of three of the lambs in Table 2. Good agreement between the qualitative and quantitative techniques is evident although there was some non-specific attachment which gave rise to relatively high levels in the anterior intestine of lamb C and in the posterior intestine of lamb D.

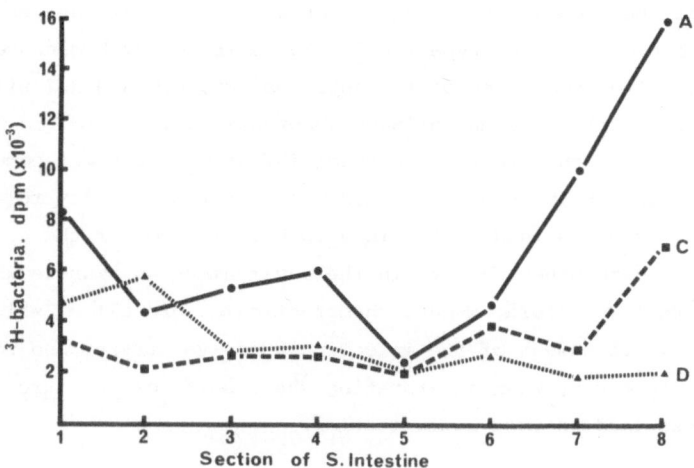

Figure 1.   Adhesion of ^{3}H-labelled K99+ E. coli to lamb brush-borders

CONCLUSIONS

The use of the brush-border adhesion test for the study of adhesive properties of E. coli has many advantages compared with other in vitro methods. Haemagglutination assays can be used but E. coli strains possessing the 987 pilus do not haemagglutinate (Isaacson et al., 1977).

There are also limitations to the use of the adhesion test. It is obvious that when looking for adhesive antigens by this means one must use brush-borders to which the bacteria producing a particular antigen will attach. It is often apparent that it is vital to use brush-borders from the host in which the organism is a potential pathogen, but even here there are certain problems viz. the areas of intestine where adhesion does not occur and therefore cannot be used for a study of the adhesive ability of E. coli strains. The variation in adhesion may be due to changes in surface receptors on the epithelial cells as they differentiate and migrate towards the villus tips. It may also indicate that susceptibility to adhesion may be age dependent.

Another consideration must also be the cultural characteristics required to enable the E. coli strain to produce the adhesive antigen. Results of tests comparing the adhesive ability and cultural conditions have resulted in the use of various media depending on the antigen under investigation. It has also been apparent that type 1 pili can mediate attachment of organisms but this attachment has not been shown to be important in the enteropathogenicity of E. coli strains. It has also been shown that the haemagglutinating properties (Old, 1972) and brush-border adhesive properties of type 1 pili are inhibited by D-mannose, whereas the adhesive properties of the antigens K88, K99 and 987 pilus are not inhibited (Sellwood, unpublished observations).

However close to the events in natural infections they may come, it should be emphasised that in vitro assays will never completely fulfill all the conditions which lead to the in vivo colonization of the intestine. There are other factors in the environment as a whole which include the normal gut flora, mucus, chemotactic factors all of which may influence the establishment of the infecting adhesive strain; and so great care is always necessary when interpreting the results of in vitro assays of the type described in this communication.

REFERENCES

Arbuckle, J.P.R., 1970. The location of Escherichia coli in the pig
    intestine. J. Med. Microbiol., 3: 333-340.
Bertschinger, H.U., Moon, H.W. and Whipp, S.C., 1972. The association of
    Escherichia coli with the small intestinal epithelium. I.
    Comparison of enteropathogenic and non-enteropathogenic porcine
    strains in pigs. Infect. Immun., 5: 595-605.
Burrows, M.R., Sellwood, R. and Gibbons, R.A., 1976. Haemagglutinating
    and adhesive properties associated with the K99 antigen of bovine
    strains of Escherichia coli. J. Gen. Microbiol., 96: 269-275.
Drees, D.T. and Waxler, G.L., 1970. Enteric colibacillosis in gnotobiotic
    swine: a fluorescent microscopic study. Am. J. Vet. Res., 31:
    1147-1157.
Duguid, J.P., Smith, W., Dempster, G. and Edmunds, P.N., 1955. Non-
    flagellar filamentous appendages ("fimbriae") and haemagglutinating
    activity in Bacterium coli. J. Path. Bact., 70: 335-348.
Evans, D.G., Silver, P., Evans, D.J.Jr., Chase, D.G. and Gorbach, S.L.,
    1973. Plasmid-controlled colonization factor associated with
    virulence in Escherichia coli enterotoxigenic for humans. Infect.
    Immun., 12: 656-667.
Gibbons, R.A., Sellwood, R., Burrows, M.R. and Hunter, P.A., 1977.
    Inheritance of resistance to neonatal E. coli diarrhoea in the pig:
    examination of the genetic system. Theor. Appl. Genet., 51: 65-70.
Isaacson, R.E., Nagy, B. and Moon, H.W., 1977. Colonization of porcine
    small intestine by Escherichia coli: colonization and adhesion
    factors of pig enteropathogens that lack K88. J. Infect. Dis., 135:
    531-539.
Jones, G.W., 1972. The adhesive properties of K88 antigen of strains of
    Escherichia coli pathogenic to neonatal pigs. Ph.D. Thesis, Univ.
    Reading, England.
Jones, G.W. and Rutter, J.M., 1972. Role of the K88 antigen in the
    pathogenesis of neonatal diarrhoea caused by Escherichia coli in
    piglets. Infect. Immun., 6: 918-927.
Jones, G.W. and Rutter, J.M., 1974. The association of K88 antigen with
    haemagglutinating activity in porcine strains of Escherichia coli.
    J. Gen. Microbiol., 84: 135-144.
Nagy, B., Moon, H.W. and Isaacson, R.E., 1976. Colonization of porcine
    small intestine by Escherichia coli: ideal colonization and adhesion
    by pig enteropathogens that lack K88 antigen and by some acapsular
    mutants. Infect. Immun., 13: 1214-1220.
Old, D.C., 1972. Inhibition of the interaction between fimbrial
    haemagglutinins and erythrocytes by D-mannose and other carbohydrates.
    J. Gen. Microbiol., 71: 149-157.
Schlechts, S. and Westphal, O., 1966. Wachstum and lipopolysaccharid-
    (O-antigen)-gehalt von Salmonellen bei zuchtung auf agarnährboden.
    Z. Bakt. Parasit., Inf. u Hyg., 200: 241-259.
Sellwood, R., Gibbons, R.A., Jones, G.W. and Rutter, J.M., 1975. Adhesion
    of enteropathogenic Escherichia coli to pig intestinal brush-borders:
    the existence of two pigs phenotypes. J. Med. Microbiol., 8: 405-411.
Sellwood, R., 1980. The interaction of the K88 antigen with porcine
    intestinal epithelial cell brush-borders. Biochim. Biophys. Acta, in
    press.

Smith, H. Williams and Linggood, M.A., 1972. Further observations on
     Escherichia coli enterotoxins with particular regard to those produced
     by atypical piglet strains and by calf and lamb strains: the
     transmissible nature of these enterotoxins and of a K antigen
     possessed by calf and lamb strains. J. Med. Microbiol., 5: 243-250.
Wilson, M.R. and Hohman, A.W., 1974. Immunity to _Escherichia coli_ in
     pigs; adhesion of enteropathogenic _Escherichia coli_ to isolated
     epithelial cells. Infect. Immun., 10: 776-782.

THE BRUSH-BORDER ADHESION TEST FOR THE ASSESSMENT OF THE ADHESIVE ABILITY
OF *ESCHERICHIA COLI* PATHOGENIC TO PIGS, CALVES AND LAMBS

Laboratory manual of the Biochemistry Department, Institute for Research
on Animal Diseases, Compton, Berkshire, England

REFERENCES

R. Sellwood, R.A. Gibbons, G.W. Jones and J.M. Rutter: Adhesion of enteropathogenic *Escherichia coli* to pig intestinal brush-borders: the
   existence of two pig phenotypes. J. Medical Microbiology <u>8</u>, 405-411,
   1975.
M.R. Burrows, R. Sellwood and R.A. Gibbons: Haemagglutinating and adhesive
   properties associated with the K99 antigen of bovine strains of
   Escherichia coli. J. Gen.Microbiol. <u>96</u>, 269-275, 1976.

The brush-border adhesion test is a test that can adequately assess the
ability of *E. coli* to attach to brush-borders prepared from the small intestine of animals which may be potential hosts for the organism and in which
it may cause diarrhoea. The method involves the preparation of brush-borders
from the small intestinal epithelial cells of the potential host; the
culturing of the coliform so that the adhesive surface antigens are produced and observation by phase contrast microscopy of attachment or no
attachment when both brush-borders and bacteria are mixed together.

1. Preparation of brush-borders

- 1 meter (approx) length of small intestine is taken from a freshly
  killed animal. (a) Pigs - any part of the small intestine will be suitable from 2 days old to an adult pig for K88 adhesion testing. The
  testing of strains possessing the 987P adhesin requires brush-borders
  prepared from the ileum of pigs. Take a 0.5 to 1 m length of intestine
  0.5 m anterior to the ileo-caecal valve. (b) Calves, lambs - 2-4 days
  old; variation in receptor distribution along the length of intestine
  will necessitate the sampling of more than one area of intestine. The
  posterior small intestine is usually suitable. Take a 1 m length of
  intestine from a freshly killed calf between 2 and 4 m anterior to the
  ileo-caecal valve.
- Intestinal contents are flushed out of the intestine with EDTA buffer
  at 20°C.
- Intestine is filled with EDTA buffer until it is slightly distended.

- Both ends of intestine are clamped using Spencer Wells forceps.
- Incubate for 30 mins at room temperature ($\sim 20^{\circ}$C).
- Discard intestinal contents and fill the intestine with half the volume of sucrose buffer at 20°C.
- Detach the epithelial cells into the fluid in the lumen of the intestine by rubbing the intestine between the fingers (2 mins).
- Collect contents of intestine.
- Centrifuge intestinal contents (10', 1000 x g) at 4°C.
- Resuspend pellet in 10-20 volumes of hypotonic EDTA solution at 4°C.
- Homogenize cell suspension with a Teflon-tipped tissue grinder (clearance 0.015-0.023 cm, A.H. Thomas Co., Philadelphia, USA) moving the pestle up and down six times whilst it is rotating at about 600 rpm.
- Centrifuge homogenate (10', 1000 x g) at 4°C.
- Resuspend pellet in hypotonic EDTA solution and repeat homogenization and centrifugation procedure discarding supernatant fluid each time and replacing with fresh hypotonic EDTA solution.
- Depending on the ability of the suspension to pellet, (this usually requires 3-4 cycles of homogenization and centrifugation) subsequent centrifugation is carried out at lower speed and for a shorter time (5 mins, 300 x g).
- When the supernatant solution is clear resuspend the pellet in 10 vols PBS solution and stand at 4°C overnight.
- Filter suspension through several layers of glass wool and centrifuge (5 mins, 300 x g).
- Repeat washing of brush-borders with PBS and resuspend to a concentration of about 1 x 10^6 brush-borders/ml counting in an improved Neubauer counting chamber. Brush-borders can be stored for long periods at -20°C after the addition of an equal volume of glycerol.

2. Bacterial cultures

- Culture *Escherichia coli* strains according to adhesive antigen under investigation.
  - (a) K88-positive strains - overnight nutrient broth at 37°C.
  - (b) K99-positive strains - overnight culture on tryptose glucose yeast extract agar (TEM) at 37°C.
  - (c) 987 piliated strains - overnight culture on Slanetz agar at 37°C.
- Centrifuge broth cultures or harvest solid agar cultures into PBS and then centrifuge (10', 1000 x g).

- Wash pellet 2 x with PBS.
- Resuspend bacteria in PBS to approximately 1×10^9 cfu/ml using the McFarland Standards Scale.

3. Adhesion test

- In a small screw-capped vial add 100 µl of brush-border suspension and 100 µl bacterial suspension.
- Mix by inverting slowly for 30 mins at room temperature.
- View a drop of suspension of phase contrast microscopy to ascertain degree of attachment.
- Use - to ++++ te denote degree of attachment.
  - no attachment to microvillus surface of brush-border; + 1 or 2 bacteria/brush-border, ++ 3-6 bacteria/brush-border, +++ 7-12 bacteria/ brush-border, ++++ 13-20 bacteria/brush-border and complete agglutination of brush-borders.

Ingredients

1) EDTA Buffer pH 6.8.

   NaCl 5.61 g, KH_2PO_4 1.09 g, Na_2HPO_4 0.795 g, KCl 0.11 g, ethylene diaminetetracetate, disodium salt (EDTA) 3.72 g, A.D. 1000 ml.

2) Sucrose Buffer pH 6.8.

   Same as above except that the EDTA was replaced by 102.6 g sucrose.

3) Hypotonic EDTA solution, pH 7.4.

   Ethylenediaminetetracetate, disodium salt (EDTA) 1.86 g, A.D. 1000 ml (pH adjusted by the addition of 0.5 M Na_2CO_3 - approx. 10 ml/litre).

4) PBS pH 7.2.

   NaCl 10 g, KCl 0.25 g, Na_2HPO_4 1.44 g, KH_2PO_4 0.25 g, A.D. 1000 ml.

5) Nutrient Broth pH 7.5.

   Lab-Lemco (Oxoid, London, U.K.) 10 g, Peptone (Difco, Detroit, USA) 10 g, NaCl 5.0 g, A.D. 1000 ml. Dissolve and sterilize at 120° for 15 mins.

6) TEM Medium.

   Lab-Lemco 5 g, bacto tryptose (Difco) 10 g, NaCl 3 g, Na_2HPO_4 $12H_2O$ 2 g, glucose 0.5 g, yeast extract (Difco) 5 g, Trace element solution[*] 5.0 ml. Adjust to pH 7.3.

   Add bacto agar (Difco) 25 g, A.D. 1000 ml. Dissolve and sterilize at

[*] Trace element solution; $FeSO_4$ $7H_2O$ 0.5 g, $ZnSO_4$ $7H_2O$ 0.5 g, $MgSO_4$ $3H_2O$ 0.5 g, 1N H_2SO_4 1.0 ml., A.D. 1000 ml.

120°C for 15 mins.

7) Slanetz Medium.

Bacto tryptose 20 g, glucose 1 g, NaCl 9 g, bacto agar 18 g, A.D. 1000 ml. Dissolve and sterilize for 15 mins.

PRELIMINARY EXPERIENCES WITH AN ENZYME-LINKED IMMUNOSORBENT ASSAY (ELISA)
FOR THE DETECTION OF THE K88 ANTIGEN OF *E. coli* IN PORCINE FAECES

P.J. van der Heijden

Central Veterinary Institute, Immunology Department, 3002 AA Rotterdam,
The Netherlands.

SUMMARY

Some preliminary experiences with a recently developed ELISA for the
detection of the K88 antigen of *E. coli* in porcine faeces are described.
Comparison of the results obtained with those of conventional bacteriological examination showed good agreement, but the ELISA was somewhat less
sensitive. The method proved to be useful for diagnosis of *E. coli* K88
associated diarrhoea on a litter basis.

INTRODUCTION

E. coli strains carrying the K88 antigen are often responsible for
neonatal and post-weaning diarrhoea in piglets. The common way to diagnose
K88 positive *E. coli* is bacteriological examination of faecal samples
followed by slide-agglutination tests. However, this is a relatively slow
method and, for large numbers of samples, also rather laborious. For these
reasons an ELISA was developed, as this technique has the advantage of
being rapid while it is easy to perform on large numbers of samples.

The principle of the ELISA for the detection of the K88 antigen of
E. coli, as well as the performance of the assay, are described in the
relating manual in these proceedings. Some additional information is presented here.

SPECIFICITY OF THE ASSAY

The anti-K88 serum used was shown to be free of antibodies against
bovine coronavirus. In the ELISA it had a low blocking titre of 1:40
against porcine rotavirus. In view of the working dilution for coating
in the K88 ELISA of 1:5,000, one can reasonably assume that the anti-rotavirus activity will be diluted out and thus will not give rise to false-
positive reactions if rotaviruses were present in the faeces.

Different strains of *Klebsiella*, *Salmonella*, *Pseudomonas* and micro-
cocci, isolated from normal as well as from diarrhoeic porcine faeces,
did not cause positive reactions in the K88 ELISA.

Several strains of *E. coli* grown *in vitro* were also tested in the ELISA. All K88 carrying strains examined gave a positive reaction; the minimum number of bacteria per ml required was 10^6 to 10^7, depending on the strain. Positive reactions were not found with *E. coli* strains lacking the K88 antigen, except for some strains possessing the K91 antigen. However, this was only observed with suspensions containing at least 10^9 bacteria per ml. Further absorption of the serum with the vaccination strain 0149:(K91):K88ac grown at $18^{\circ}C$, did not result in a decrease of the observed cross-reactivity. In practice it is unlikely that concentrations of $\geq 10^9$ bacteria per ml of *E. coli* strains possessing the K91 antigen, but lacking the K88 antigen, will occur in the faeces of piglets. Nevertheless, attempts are now being made to prepare mono-specific antisera against K88 with the aid of *E. coli* strain K12:K88.

At present it is advisable to incorporate a specificity check into each ELISA plate, especially when no other diagnostic techniques are used in parallel. There are several possibilities for specificity checks, for example coating with negative serum, incorporation of standard positive and negative faecal samples, or a blocking test as employed in our institute in the ELISA for the detection of bovine rotavirus (these proceedings). In the K88 ELISA we use standard negative and positive faecal samples. A blocking test is not employed for two reasons. First, we compared the results of ELISA and conventional bacteriological techniques with 55 faecal samples from diarrhoeic and healthy piglets (Table 1). As can be seen only two samples were scored positive by ELISA that were not confirmed by bacteriological examination. Secondly, since the test is used for diagnosis on a litter basis, large numbers of samples obtained during each outbreak are examined. Incorporation of a blocking step would diminish the capacity of the assay and delay the results obtained. In view of the results shown in table 1, such a blocking step does not appear necessary as it is not likely to influence the diagnosis.

SENSITIVITY OF THE ASSAY

The results shown on table 1 suggest that the K88 ELISA is somewhat less sensitive than the conventional bacteriological procedure. However, so far a number of outbreaks of diarrhoea in different herds, both in neonatal and in post-weaning pigs, could easily be diagnosed by obtaining faecal samples from several pigs in each litter.

CONCLUSION

The first results obtained with the K88 ELISA show that the test can be used for diagnosis on a litter or herd basis. Further work is in progress to improve the specificity and sensitivity of the test in order to be able to reduce the number of samples that have to be examined from each outbreak to arrive at a reliable diagnosis.

Table 1. Comparison of ELISA and conventional bacteriological examination for K88 positive *E. coli* in porcine faeces.

		ELISA	
		+	–
Bacteriological examination	+	31	7
	–	2	15

ENZYME-LINKED IMMUNOSORBENT ASSAY (ELISA) FOR THE DETECTION OF THE K88
ANTIGEN OF *ESCHERICHIA COLI* IN PORCINE FAECES

Laboratory manual of the Central Veterinary Institute, Immunology Department, 3002 AA Rotterdam, The Netherlands.

P.J. van der Heijden

PRINCIPLE OF THE ASSAY

A polystyrene solid phase is coated with antibody directed against the
K88 antigen of *E. coli*. During incubation of the coated surface with a
faecal extract, antigen (if present) will be caught by specific antibody.
This antigen can be labeled with antibody covalently linked to the enzyme
horseradish peroxidase (conjugate). The bound conjugate can be visualized
by the addition of a chromogenic substrate.

PREPARATION OF GOAT ANTI *E. coli* K88 SERUM

E. coli 0149:(K91):K88ac, grown on serum agar plates at 37°C during 18
h, are harvested in 0.15% formaldehyde in 0.01 M PBS pH 7.5 and incubated
at room temperature during 30 min. The bacteria are washed twice in the
same buffer without formaldehyde and a suspension of approximately 5.10^{7}
bacteria/ml is prepared. A volume of 2.5 ml of this suspension is mixed
with an equal volume of a 2% aluminium hydroxide gel. After stirring during
1.5 h, the mixture is emulsified in 5 ml of Freund's incomplete adjuvant.

A goat is injected with volumes of 1.5 ml at three different sites,
i.e. intramuscularly (i.m.) in both hind legs and subcutaneously in the
neck. After 21 days this procedure is repeated with a freshly prepared
bacterial suspension adsorbed onto aluminium hydroxide gel; a last injection is given i.m. with killed bacteria ten days later. Blood is withdrawn
seven days after the last injection. The serum is made specific by repeated
absorption with the above *E. coli* strain grown at 18°C. Specificity is
checked by slide-agglutination (manual in these proceedings) with the
vaccination strain grown at 18 and at 37°C, and with pathogenic *E. coli*
strains lacking the K88 antigen.

SEPARATION OF IgG FROM GOAT ANTI K88 SERUM

IgG is precipitated by addition of saturated $(NH_4)_2SO_4$ solution to a
concentration of 35%. The mixture is allowed to stand overnight at 4°C.

After centrifugation (2,800 g, 20 min, 4°C) the precipitate is washed once
with 50% $(NH_4)_2SO_4$ and dissolved in PBS. After dialysis overnight against
the same buffer, the IgG suspension is centrifuged (2,800 g, 20 min, 4°C)
and the supernatant is stored at -20°C.

PREPARATION OF THE CONJUGATE AND THE SUBSTRATE SOLUTION

The conjugate and the substrate solution are prepared as described
in the ELISA manual of the Central Veterinary Institute, The Netherlands
for the detection of bovine rotavirus (these proceedings).

PREPARATION OF STANDARD ANTIGEN

A formaldehyde killed suspension of *E. coli* 0149:(K91):K88ac is washed once with PBS. After centrifugation (1,000 g, 15 min, 4°C) the bacteria
are suspended in PBS and homogenized by ultrasonic treatment (MSE, 3 x 5
sec, maximum power) and then centrifuged at 2,800 g during 20 min at 4°C.
The supernatant is used as standard antigen and stored at 4°C (no loss of
activity has been found after six months at this temperature).

PREPARATION OF FAECAL HOMOGENATES

Faecal samples are mixed with an equal volume of ELISA-buffer and homogenized on a Vortex mixer. The samples are treated ultrasonically (MSE, 3 x
5 sec, maximum power), particulate material is removed by centrifugation
(400 g, 10 min), and the supernatant is used in the test. Storage, if
necessary, is at 4°C).

PERFORMANCE OF THE ASSAY

- Coat polystyrene plates (Cooke, Dynatech microtiter, M 129A) with 100 µl
  volumes of an appropriate dilution of goat anti K88 IgG in coating buffer
  overnight at 37°C. The optimal dilution is determined by checkerboard
  titration as described in the manual of the rotavirus ELISA of our
  institute (these proceedings).
  After coating the plates can be stored at -20°C for at least four months.
- Wash the plates thoroughly by nine showers with 0.05% Tween 80 in demineralized water.
- Fill the wells of row 1 with 100 µl volumes of ELISA buffer. Prepare in
  row 2 a two-fold dilution series of the standard antigen suspension
  (final volumes of 100 µl). Fill the wells of row 3 with 100 µl volumes
  of known negative faecal homogenates diluted 1:2 and 1:5. Fill the re-

maining wells with similar volumes and dilutions of test samples, using
two wells for each dilution (one in two dilutions are prepared by adding
50 µl volumes of test samples and equal volumes of ELISA-buffer; 1:5
dilutions by adding 20 and 80 µl, respectively).

- Incubate for 2 h at 37°C.
- Wash the plates thoroughly by nine showers with 0.05% Tween 80 in
  demineralized water.
- Add to each well volumes of 100 µl conjugate at an appropriate dilution
  in ELISA-buffer containing 1% bovine serum albumin (BSA, Fraction V,
  Baker). The optimal dilution is determined by checkerboard titration
  as described in the manual of the rotavirus ELISA of our institute
  (these proceedings).
- Incubate for 1 h at 37°C;
- Wash thoroughly by nine showers with 0.05% Tween 80 in demineralized
  water.
- Add to each well volumes of 100 µl of the substrate solution.
- Incubate 40 min at room temperature and stop the reaction by adding 25 µl
  0.1% NaN_3 solution.
- Read the test by the naked eye or by Titertek^R Multiskan.
  The test is accepted if the titre of the standard positive antigen suspension is normal and if the samples in row 3 prove to be negative. Test
  samples are scored positive if both the colour in the well containing the
  1:2 dilution and that in the well containing the 1:5 dilution, is more
  intensive than the colour of the well containing the last positive
  dilution of the standard antigen (for details see the manual of the rotavirus ELISA of our institute).

MEDIA AND BUFFERS
Serum agar pH 7.5
2% Difco-agar (Difco, 0140-01)
1% Bacto-Pepton (Difco, 0118-05)
0.5% NaCl (Baker)
10% Horse serum
PBS pH 7.5
$Na_2HPO_4 \cdot 2H_2O$	1.6 gr
KH_2PO_4	0.14 gr
NaCl	8.5 gr

Aqua dest. ad 1000 ml

ELISA BUFFER

Solution A: 0.5 M NaCl

0.01 M $Na_2HPO_4 \cdot 2H_2O$

0.05 % Tween 80

500 ml aqua dest.

Solution B: 0.5 M NaCl

0.01 M KH_2PO_4

0.05% Tween 80

500 ml aqua dest.

Adjust the pH of solution A to pH 7.5 with solution B.

COATING BUFFER

Solution A: $NaHCO_3$ 2.1 gr

aqua dest.   500 ml

Solution B: Na_2CO_3 2.7 gr

aqua dest.   500 ml

Adjust the pH of solution A to pH 9.6 with solution B.

Hydrophobic interaction chromatography

Laboratory manual of the Department of Bacteriology and Epizootology
Swedish University of Agricultural Sciences, College of Veterinary Medicine,
Biomedicum, Box 583, S-751 23 Uppsala, Sweden.

Reference: C.J. Smyth, P. Jonsson, E. Olsson, O. Söderlind, J. Rosengren,
S. Hjertén and T. Wadström: Differences in hydrophobic surface characteristics of porcine enteropathogenic Escherichia coli with and without K88
antigen as revealed by hydrophobic interaction chromatography. Infect
Immun 22: 462-472, 1978.

Hydrophobic interaction chromatography (HIC) is a procedure based on the
hydrophobic interaction between nonpolar groups on a gel and nonpolar
regions of a solute, e.g. of a protein. Adsorbents with alkyl or aryl substituents linked to agarose gels have been synthesized. The degree of
hydrophobicity of the substituents and the degree of substitution can be
varied.

A standard test procedure for measuring surface hydrophobicity of bacteria,
using commercially available hydrophobic gels, has been developed with
enterotoxigenic E coli (ETEC) isolated from neonatal diarrhoea. ETEC
assayed for heat-labile (LT) and heat-stable enterotoxin (ST) are also
assayed for protein surface structures (so called colonization factors:
synonym adhesins) such as K88 and K99 antigens. HIC is used to reveal
these antigens or other potential adhesins.

1. Hydrophobic gels

Phenyl Sepharose CL4B(R) and Octyl Sepharose CL4B(R) are purchased from
Pharmacia Fine Chemicals, Uppsala, Sweden.

2. Preparation of bacterial suspensions

X)

Strains are grown in 100 ml of a tryptone-yeast extract medium (TY-1)
which contains 1% (wt/vol) glucose in 1-litre indented shake flasks
(120 rpm; 37°C, for 1 to 2 h) to an absorbance at 600 nm (A_{600}) of 1.0 in
a 10-mm light path, corresponding to about 1.4×10^9 colony-forming units
(CFU) per ml. Inocula comprised 10 ml of 16- to 18-h cultures grown under
identical growth conditions in TY-1 medium. Portions of test cultures (20ml)
were centrifuged (4,000 x g; 10 min; 20°C), and cell pellets were gently
suspended in 4 M sodium chloride or 1 M ammonium sulfate buffered with
10 mM sodium phosphate buffer (pH 6.8) to obtain homogeneous suspensions of
about 2×10^{10} to 4×10^{10} bacteria per ml.

3. Hydrophobic interaction chromatography (HIC)

Hydrophobic gels were washed extensively with buffered 4 M sodium chloride
or 1 M ammonium sulfate to remove fine particles. Gel suspensions were
allowed to equilibrate at 20 to 24°C, and chromatography was performed at
the same temperature. Columns comprised short-ended glass Pasteur pipettes
(internal diameter, 5 mm; length 85 mm), plugged with a little glass wool
and fitted with clamped Teflon tubing. Gel beds were packed to a height of
30 mm (ca. 0.6 ml gel bed volume) by gravity feed and washed with 10 ml of
buffered 4 M sodium chloride or 1 M ammonium sulfate. Bacterial suspensions

(100 µl, 2×10^9 to 4×10^9 bacteria) were allowed to drain into the gel beds. Gel beds were washed with 5 ml of buffered 4 M sodium chloride or 1 M ammonium sulfate (flow rate 1 to 2 ml/min).

4. Evaluation of HIC test results

For routine purposes (e.g., screening of hydrophobicity of strains), visual comparison of the opacity of the eluate with an appropriately diluted 100-µl portion of the original suspension was used to assess the degree of adsorption. Visible adsorption to the gel bed and its appearance were recorded.

5. Desorption of bacteria from HIC gels

Release of adsorbed bacteria was obtained by washing the gel bed with 10 ml of the 10 mM sodium phosphate buffer (pH 6.8). The turbidities of eluates were again compared visually with appropriately diluted portions of the original suspensions. Adsorption and desorption were also quantified by viable counts and bacterial counts related to measurements of A_{600} of suspensions in a 10-mm light path.

6. Determination of bacterial concentrations

(i) Standard curves were constructed relating measurements of A_{600} in a 10 mm light path to CFU of bacteria per ml. This was done by using a K88 antigen positive (K88+) ETEC strain grown to mid-logarithmic phase in TY-1 medium. (It must be emphasized that A_{600} increases markedly for identical suspensions of both K88+ and K88− E coli in concentrations of sodium chloride 0.3 M. It is, thus, important to dilute suspensions or column eluates with the diluent or eluant relevant to particular experiments.)

(ii) Viable counts. Bacterial suspensions were diluted ten-fold in 0.15 M sodium chloride buffered with 10 mM sodium phosphate buffer (pH 6.8). Eighteen 25-µl drops (MLA micropipette, Vernon, N.Y., with sterile disposable tips) for each appropriate dilution were applied to surface-dried heart infusion agar plates (six per plate), and CFU were counted after incubation at 37°C for 24 h.

7. Controls

ETEC strains with K88 and K99 antigens should be grown at 18°C in the TY-1 medium. The formation of these two and other adhesins (CFA/I and CFA/II in human ETEC strains) will be suppressed at this suboptimal temperature, i.e. the strains should be HIC negative. Such HIC− bacteria are recovered in the effluent while the same strain grown at 37°C will express the adhesin and bind (HIC positive) and can be eluted by washing the gel columns as described under desorption (point 5 above)

Interpretation of test results

ETEC strains which bind to Octyl or Phenyl Sepharose under these conditions (HIC+ strains) should be tested for K88, K99 and 987P adhesins by agglutination and/or haemagglutination (HA) tests. Strains which do not react with these sera should be subjected to O:H serotyping (strains with a deficient LPS, ie. rough strains may behave as HIC$^+$ strain). HIC$^+$ strains should also be subjected to brush border adhesion tests according to a separate manual. Strains (K88$^-$, K99$^-$, and 987P$^-$) which adhere to brush border preparations should be further investigated by electron microscopy for adhesins of pilus nature or filamentous-like structures.

X) TY-1 Medium

The medium consists of the following ingridients in grams per litre:

Tryptone (Difco) 10g; Yeast extract (Difco) 5g; D-glucose, 10g (sterilise separately and add into the cold sterilised medium);NH_4Cl, 2,5g; $Na_2HPO_4 \cdot 2H_2$, 15g; KH_2PO_4, 6g; $Na_2SO_4 \cdot 10H_2O$, 0.5g; $MgSO_4 \cdot 7H_2O$, 0.2g; Trace elem. soln. 1ml, (sterilised separately and add into the cold medium); Distilled water 1.000ml; Adjust pH to 7.2 and sterilise by autoclaving at 120°C for 15 minutes.

Trace elements:

$CaCl_2 \cdot 2H_2O$, 0.5g; FeCl, $\cdot$ 6H$_2$0. 16.7g; $ZnSO_4 \cdot 7H_2O$, 0.18g ;$CuSO_4 \cdot 5HO$, 0.16g; $MnSO_4 \cdot 4H_2O$, 0.15g; $CoCl_2 \cdot 6H_2O$. 0.18g; sodium-EDTA 20.1g; distilled water 1.000 ml.

MIXED DIARRHOEAL INFECTION IN CALVES: THE RELATIVE IMPORTANCE OF 2
INTERACTING ENTEROPATHOGENS

Saul Tzipori

'Attwood' Veterinary Research Laboratory, Melbourne, Australia and
Moredun Research Institute, 408 Gilmerton Road, Edinburgh EH17 7JH

ABSTRACT

Some of the causes of neonatal diarrhoea in suckling calves aged up
to 10 weeks were examined.   The susceptibility of calves to the diarrhoea-inducing effect of calf rotavirus was found to be age dependent.
Calves over 6 days old were resistant to clinical diarrhoea although they
did excrete virus in their faeces and subsequently developed antibody to
rotavirus.   An enterotoxigenic $E.$ $coli$ (ETEC) inoculated orally into
either gnotobiotic or suckling calves aged $1\frac{1}{2}$ to 26 days did not cause
diarrhoea.   In contrast, diarrhoea was consistently produced in gnotobiotic and suckling calves between one and 15 days of age when they were
inoculated with both calf rotavirus and ETEC.   In general, diarrhoea
appeared after a rotavirus incubation period of approximately 3 days and
was independent of the order in which the 2 microbial agents were given.

INTRODUCTION

Diarrhoea in calves is one of the most important causes of neonatal
mortality.   The disease remains largely uncontrolled because of its complex aetiology.   As well as different infectious agents, immunological,
nutritional and environmental factors are also involved in precipitating
the disease.   Microorganisms most commonly encountered in field investigations of diarrhoea are enterotoxigenic $E.$ $coli$ (ETEC) and rotavirus
(Acres et al, 1977).   The role of rotavirus as a cause of diarrhoea in
calves and other mammals has been extensively reviewed (Holmes, 1979).

Preliminary work has shown that calves are clinically susceptible to
rotavirus infections only for the first few days of life.   In the
field, on the other hand, rotavirus often appears to be associated with
diarrhoea in calves up to 10 weeks old.   In this study a field outbreak
of diarrhoea was examined to determine which other infectious or non-
infectious factors act in combination with rotavirus in precipitating
the disease.

MATERIALS AND METHODS

Case history - Outbreaks of diarrhoea have occurred over the last few
years in a 400 suckled beef herd in Victoria, Australia.   In 1978 most

of the 400 newborn calves developed diarrhoea.   Nine of the 11 faecal
samples collected from scouring calves contained rotavirus (isolate C6)
and 3 of them had 1 or 2, stable toxin-producing ETEC organisms   (O20:
K106:K99$^+$)

Experimental animals - The calves used for these experiments were either
gnotobiotic (17 calves), colostrum deprived (7 calves) or suckling (16
calves).

Viruses - Calf rotavirus isolates C1, C3 and C4 (Tzipori et al, 1980) were
used for experiment 1 while C6, the rotavirus isolated from the field
outbreak was used for the remaining 5 experiments.   A fifteen ml aliquot
of faecal filtrates containing C6 was used as the standard oral inoculum
for each calf.   The presence of virus in faeces was determined by
electron microscopy.

Bacteria - Four ml of tryptose soya broth containing 10^6 to 10^8 organisms,
serotype O20:K106:K99$^+$ were used as standard ETEC oral inoculum per calf.
ETEC organisms in the faeces were identified by their O antigen and were
tested for K99 by the slide agglutination test.

Serology - A complement fixation (CF) test was used to estimate circu-
lating antibody titres against rotavirus using the tissue culture adapted
monkey rotavirus SA11 as antigen.

RESULTS

Experiment 1 - Seven gnotobiotic (GB) and 5 colostrum deprived (CD)
calves, aged between 1 and 10 days, were inoculated with one of 4 calf
rotavirus isolates.   Experimental inoculation of calves with rotavirus
induced diarrhoea in calves less than 7 days old.   Calves 7 days old or
older developed subclinical rotavirus infections only.   All 12 calves
developed complement fixing (CF) antibody against rotavirus.

Experiment 2 -   Two CD and 4 GB calves aged between 2 hours and 26 days
were inoculated with ETEC.   Diarrhoea was evident only in 2 calves less
than 24 hours of age.   One 36 hour calf passed loose but not diarrhoeic
faeces.   Older calves showed no symptoms although they excreted the
organism in their faeces.

Experiment 3 - Four GB calves aged between 8 and 13 days were inoculated
with rotavirus and ETEC at short intervals (Table 1).   Three calves

developed diarrhoea that lasted 3 to 4 days and excreted both organisms in their faeces. One calf, although dosed twice with rotavirus, failed to become infected and developed neither diarrhoea nor CF antibody against rotavirus.

TABLE 1 - THE RESPONSE OF GNOTOBIOTIC CALVES TO ORAL INOCULATION WITH ENTEROTOXIGENIC E. COLI AND ROTAVIRUS

Age at Inoculation (Days)		Clinical Diarrhoea		Shedding	
Rotavirus	E. coli	Incubation (Days)	Duration (Days)	Virus	E. coli
8	11	0.5 h	4	+	++
9	13	1	3	+	+
9	13	-	-	-	+
12	10	3	4	+	+

Experiment 4 - Four suckling calves aged between 3 and 10 days were inoculated with ETEC and 4 others aged between 6 and 10 days were inoculated with rotavirus. As with CD and GB calves, the suckling calves showed no evidence of diarrhoea to either of the two agents (Table 2). One calf inoculated with rotavirus passed solid creamy-white faeces for 1 day. The 2 calves that showed evidence of sub-clinical infection with rotavirus had lower pre-inoculation CF antibody titres (8 and < 2 respectively) than the other 2 in the group (64 and 32)

TABLE 2 - INOCULATION OF SUCKLING CALVES WITH EITHER ROTAVIRUS OR ENTEROTOXIGENIC E. COLI

Age at Inoculation		Clinical Diarrhoea		Shedding		Rotavirus CF antibody	
Virus	E.coli	Incubation (Days)	Duration (Days)	Virus	E.coli	Pre- inoculation	Post-
-	3	-	-	-	+	128	64
-	4	-	-	-	+	128	32
-	9	-	-	-	+	64	32
-	10	-	-	-	+	32	64
6	-	-	-	-	-	64	128
8	-	3	1*	+	-	8	64
10	-	-	-	+	-	< 2	16
10	-	-	-	-	-	32	16

*Calf passed creamy-white faeces for 1 day

Experiment 5 - Eight suckling calves aged between 5 and 15 days were inoculated with ETEC and rotavirus either simultaneously or at short intervals. (Table 3). The incubation period varied between 2 and 5 days and diarrhoea lasted 5 to 6 days in calves that were not killed earlier. There was no difference in the length of the incubation period and the severity of the diarrhoea between calves with high and low pre-inoculation CF antibody titres against rotavirus.

TABLE 3 - INOCULATIONS OF SUCKLING CALVES WITH BOTH ROTAVIRUS AND ENTEROTOXIGENIC E. COLI

Age at Inoculation		Clinical Diarrhoea		Shedding		CF Antibody	
Virus	E.coli	Incubation (Days)	Duration (Days)	Virus	E. coli	Pre- Inoculation	Post-
5	5	3	5	+	++	512	128
7	7	3	4*	+	+	< 2	< 2
9	9	3	1*	+	+	64	8
12	12	5	5	+	+	512	64
14	14	2	1*	+	+	64	16
15	15	3	6	+	+	64	16
13	9	4	5	+	+	256	32
14	10	3	5	+	+	16	8

* Calf killed

Generally, in combined infections with ETEC and rotavirus, the disease appeared approximately 3 days after the rotavirus inoculations and was independent of which of the 2 microorganisms was given first (Tables 1 and 3). Furthermore, the disease coincided more closely with faecal excretion of rotavirus rather than of ETEC. Infections with ETEC usually became established within 24 hours of inoculation and bacterial shedding in the faeces fluctuated considerably over a much longer period than rotavirus excretion.

DISCUSSION

Calves 7 days old and older appear to be resistant to the diarrhoea-inducing effect of the 4 rotavirus isolates used. Calves older than 7 days showed evidence of sub-clinical infection followed by sero-conversion. It was shown too that the ETEC used for these experiments was capable of inducing diarrhoea in calves less than 24 hours old. Similar observations were made previously by others (Smith and Hall, 1967).

The inoculation of GB or suckling calves with both agents, simultaneously or at certain intervals, induced diarrhoea which was independent
of age. The diarrhoeal illness resembled that observed in the field
outbreak where the 2 microorganisms used in these experiments were
isolated. This experimental work can be considered a reconstruction of
the disease outbreak seen in the field. Frequently ETEC could not be
detected in faeces and when present only small numbers could be isolated.
As we have examined larger numbers of colonies per sample (10 colonies)
than most other investigators we concluded that their presence and
significance in the past may have been overlooked.

The interpretation of post-inoculation CF antibody titres was
difficult as no distinction could be made between that produced by the
calf or acquired from colostrum. While high level of CF antibody
against rotavirus appeared to be effective in preventing infections with
rotavirus alone (Table 2), in dual infections it had little effect in
preventing either infection or diarrhoea. To date, microbial agents
that have been associated with diarrhoea in young calves include ETEC,
rotavirus, coronavirus, cryptosporidia and possibly astrovirus and
Newbury agent or calicivirus. We have demonstrated that the con-
currence of two of the above listed organisms can precipitate a disease
in circumstances where each one acting independently may not. It is
likely that there are many more combinations which would induce a
disease with the severity depending partly on other non-infectious contributing factors. Only field investigations involving a sequential
examination of material for viral, bacterial and protozoan enteropathogens, as well as other non-infectious factors, would lead to a
correct diagnosis. It is no wonder that vaccines developed to combat
only one enteric agent have been singularly ineffective in controlling
diarrhoea in young domestic animals.

REFERENCES

1. Acres, S.D., Saunders, J.R. and Radostits, O.M. Acute undiffer-
      entiated neonatal diarrhoea of beef calves: the prevalence of
      enterotoxigenic E. coli reo-like (rota) virus and other
      enteropathogens in cow-calf herds. Canadian Vet. J. 18,
      113-121 (1977).

2. Holmes, I.H. Viral gastroenteritis. Prog. Med. Virol. 25, 1-36,
      1979.

3. Tzipori, S., Making, T. and Smith, M.   The clinical response of
    gnotobiotic calves, pigs and lambs to inoculations with human,
    calf, pig and foal rotavirus isolates.   Aust. J. Exp. Med.
    Biol. Sc. 58, (in press) 1980.

4. Smith, H.W. and Hall, S.   Observations by the ligated intestine
    segment and oral inoculation methods on E. coli.   Infection
    in pigs, calves, lambs and rabbits.   J. Path. Bact. 93,
    499-529 (1967.

PIGLET ENTERITIS; FIELD AND LABORATORY EVALUATION OF ENTEROPATHOGENS ASSOCIATED WITH 3 DISEASE ENTITIES

Saul Tzipori

Attwood Veterinary Research Laboratory, Westmeadows

Melbourne 3047, Australia

ABSTRACT

The aetiology and pathogenesis of 3 diarrhoeal disease entities were investigated in intensive piggeries and in the laboratory. These include, early neonatal diarrhoea occurring in 8 to 16 hour old piglets, neonatal diarrhoea affecting piglets from 3 days to 3 or 4 week old, and postweaning diarrhoea affecting 3 to 4 week old, newly weaned piglets. The role of rotavirus which was found to be involved at some stage with each disease entity, was evaluated.

INTRODUCTION

There are now many reports describing field and experimental studies on rotavirus infection in piglets. Pig rotavirus has been shown to produce severe diarrhoeal illness in gnotobiotic and colostrum deprived piglets. The virus is widespread and there is no suggestion of virulence variation. This study examines the role of rotavirus in the pathogenesis of 3 diarrhoeal disease entities recognised now in Australian piggeries.

(a) Early neonatal diarrhoea - in mid-1977 severe outbreaks of diarrhoea in suckling piglets occurred almost simultaneously in 3 large intensive piggeries (Tzipori et al., 1980a). The disease was characterised by the onset of diarrhoea within the first 12 hours of life. Affected piglets were dirty, depressed, inactive and dehydrated. Response to treatment was poor. Histological sections of gut from sick animals revealed little change apart from evidence of bacterial adherence. Three serotypes of non-haemolytic enterotoxogenic E. coli (ETEC), were isolated. These include O20: KNT:HNM: K88[+], O64: KV142: HNM: K88[+] and O8:K85ab: HNM: K99[+]. All 3 are stable toxin producers. No viruses were observed in faeces examined by electron microscopy, or isolated by inoculations of faecal filtrates into gnotobiotic piglets. Affected piglets in these piggeries either died within 24 hours, recovered after 24 hours, or continued to scour for 3 to 4 days and then died.   Only faeces from piglets with protracted diarrhoea invariably contained rotavirus.   A similar disease was induced in newborn gnotobiotic piglets by all 3 ETEC serogroups;   there was evidence of bacterial adherence to enterocytes, but little or no histological and enzymological change.

(b)   Neonatal diarrhoea - outbreaks of diarrhoea occurring from 3 days of age to weaning of 3- to 4-week-old piglets, had often been associated with excretions of rotavirus in the faeces with or without ETEC.   The ability of pig rotavirus to induce diarrhoea was examined in gnotobiotic, artificially reared or conventional 4 day old piglets derived from the same litter (Tzipori and Williams, 1978).   Four successive passages of the virus in gnotobiotic piglets induced severe diarrhoea within 20 to 24 hours of administration.   The diarrhoea lasted several days causing dehydration loss of weight and some deaths.   Newborn litters of piglets were left to be suckled for 36 hours after which half of them were taken away and artificially reared on reconstituted evaporated cows milk.   The suckling piglets developed little or no diarrhoea when inoculated with rotavirus, whereas artificially reared piglets developed moderate to severe diarrhoea with few deaths.

TABLE 1 - EXPERIMENTAL INFECTION OF PIGLETS WITH ROTAVIRUS AT 4 DAYS OF AGE - LITTER A

Item	Group No. and Treatment	Incubation Period (Days)	Duration of Diarrhoea (Days)	Fate	Virus Detected
		3	1	recovered	+
		3	1	"	+
Suckling	1	3	1	"	+
	inoculated	...	...	...	
		3	...	killed	+
		1	8	recovered	+
	2	1	4	"	
Artificially	inoculated	1	7	died	+
reared		1	7	"	+
	3	...	...	...	...
	control	...	...	...	...

TABLE 2 - EXPERIMENTAL INFECTION OF PIGLETS WITH ROTAVIRUS AT 4 DAYS OF AGE - LITTER B

Item	Group No. and Treatment	Incubation Period (Days)	Duration of Diarrhoea (Days)	Fate	Virus Detected
Suckling	1	...	...	...	-
	inoculated	...	...	...	-
		...	...	...	-
		2	4	recovered	+
Artificially	2	3	1.5	"	+
reared	inoculated	3.5	0.5	"	+
		3	4	"	+
	3	...	...	...	-
	control	...	...	...	-

Seven to 10 days old suckling piglets that showed no clinical illness when exposed to either pig rotavirus or non-haemolytic ETEC alone developed severe diarrhoea when inoculated simultaneously with pig rotavirus and ETEC. (c) Postweaning diarrhoea (PWD) - it has been known for some time that ETEC are the primary cause of PWD.   However, recently rotavirus was implicated (Woode et al., 1975; Bohl et al., 1978).   In one piggery, some aspects of PWD during the first week after early weaning were investigated.   A haemolytic (H) ETEC strain 0149: K91: H10: K88[+] was regularly recovered from piglets with PWD, while rotavirus was demonstrated on a number of occasions.   Prior to weaning, piglets were almost free of H ETEC.   Five to 7 days after weaning all were shedding H ETEC.   The role of rotavirus in PWD was unclear.   After birth, the decline of maternal neutralising antibody to rotavirus coincided with the immediate postweaning period (3 to 5 weeks after birth).   This was followed by an increase in antibody levels, 5 to 8 weeks after birth.   The H ETEC and the rotavirus isolated from the piggery were studied in 4-week old gnotobiotic piglets.   Piglets fed on milk diet were found to be extremely susceptible to the H ETEC, less susceptible to the infection immediately after change of diet from milk to dry food, and were almost completely resistant 4 days after the change to dry food.   There was no difference in clinical response when piglets were fed either high or low energy weaner diet.   Piglets fed milk showed mild symptoms of diarrhoea when inoculated with rotavirus; more severe symptoms when inoculated immediately after change of diet from milk to dry food, and complete resistance when inoculated 4 days after the change.   Under the conditions of these experiments the H ETEC induced more serious disease in 4-week-old gnotobiotic piglets than the rotavirus.   Infection of piglets with both agents given sequentially produced diarrhoeal disease that was more severe than that induced by each agent separately.   In the presence of rotavirus infection, the period of postweaning susceptibility to H ETEC was longer than 4 days following the change to dry food (Tzipori et al., 1980b).

CONCLUSION

Although pig rotavirus induces severe diarrhoea and sometimes death in colostrum-deprived, 1- to 20-day-old piglets, suckling piglets appear to be well protected against the adverse effects of infection.   The presence of rotavirus was demonstrated at some stage in each of the 3 disease entities examined (a, b, c).   In our opinion rotavirus played little or no role in disease a, perhaps had a more prominent role but definitely depended on a 'contributing factor' e.g. presence of ETEC in b, and may have potentiated the postweaning diarrhoea caused primarily by H ETEC in C.   The presence of enteropathogens at weaning however is only partially responsible, it is the abrupt change of diet and the effect it has on the physiology of the gut that precipitates the disease.

REFERENCES

Bohl, E.H., Kohler, E.M., Saif, L.J., Cross, R.F., Angus, A.G. and Theil, K.W.: Rotavirus as a cause of diarrhoea in pigs.   J.A.V.M.A. 172: 458-463, 1978.

Tzipori, S. and Williams, H.F.: diarrhoea in piglets inoculated with rotavirus.   Aust. Vet. J. 172: 188-192, 1978.

Tzipori, S., Jones, R.T. and Fahey, V.A.: Early neonatal diarrhoea of piglets associated with non-haemolytic enterotoxigenic E. Coli. Aust. Vet. J. 56: 154-155, 1980.

Tzipori, S., Chandler, D., Smith, M. and Makin, T.: Infections of 4-week old gnotobiotic piglets with E. Coli or rotavirus and feed milk or dry food.   Aust. Vet. J. 56: 1980 (in press)

Woode, G.N., Bridger, J., Hall, G.A., Jones, I.M. and Jackson, G.; The isolation of reovirus-like agents (rotavirus) from acute gastro-enteritis of piglets. J. Med. Microbiol. 9: 203-209, 1976.

CRYPTOSPORIDIOSIS IN CALVES: SIGNIFICANCE WITHIN THE ENTERITIS SYNDROME AND DIAGNOSIS OF INFECTION

S. Tzipori and K.W. Angus

Moredun Research Institute, 408 Gilmerton Road, Edinburgh, Scotland

ABSTRACT

Two field outbreaks of calf diarrhoea attributed to cryptosporidiosis are described. The epidemiology and clinical manifestations of the disease in one herd is outlined. The life-cycle of the parasite, and the diagnosis, histopathological lesions and significance of the disease produced in experimentally-infected lambs are discussed.

INTRODUCTION

The protozoon cryptosporidium has been known since the beginning of the century. It has been reported in mammals, birds and reptiles, and appears to have world-wide distribution (Levine, 1973). It is believed to be host-specific and to have a life-cycle similar to that of other enteric coccidia. Cryptosporidia differ from other coccidia in that they are extracellular organisms which adhere to the microvillous borders of enterocytes.

Direct association between cryptosporidia and outbreaks of diarrhoea in calves was confirmed only recently, when field evidence suggested that they might be important pathogens (Pohlenz et al, 1978; Snodgrass et al, 1980; Tzipori et al, 1980). Of four field outbreaks of calf diarrhoea investigated in recent months in Scotland, two were attributed solely to cryptosporidium infection, while a third was attributed to mixed infections including cryptosporidium. Faecal homogenates containing cryptosporidium oocysts but no other known enteropathogenic agent induced diarrhoea in an experimentally-inoculated 9 day-old calf. Diagnosis of infection was made by identifying oocysts in faeces, and by histological examination of the gut.

FIELD CASES

The first outbreak occurred in a housed herd of 41 suckling beef calves born over a period of 8 weeks. Thirty-five calves had mild to moderate diarrhoea, the more severe cases being in younger animals. The youngest affected calf was 5 days, the oldest 39 days old. Eight cases of diarrhoea relapsed within 3-4 weeks after the initial episodes. Faeces were examined for enterotoxigenic *Escherichia coli* and enteric

viruses, but none was detected (Tzipori et al, 1980). Eighteen diarrhoeic calves were excreting cryptosporidium oocysts, but none was seen in
faeces from non-diarrhoeic calves. In a second beef herd, 16 faeces
samples (12 from diarrhoeic calves, 4 from non-diarrhoeic calves) were
examined for enteropathogenic agents. Eleven of the 12 samples from
diarrhoeic calves contained cryptosporidium oocysts, but none was found
in the remaining samples. No other known enteropathogen was detected.

LIFE-CYCLE

The life-cycle of cryptosporidium was investigated in guinea pigs
(Vetterling et al, 1971) and calves (Pohlenz et al, 1978). An asexual or
schizogonic cycle with 2 generations of schizonts containing 8 and 4
merozoites respectively, is followed by a sexual cycle in which macro-
gametes, microgametocytes and zygotes develop. Infection is thought to
follow ingestion of oocysts, each containing 4 sporozoites.

DIAGNOSIS

Experimental infections of calves and lambs indicate that there is
close correlation between diarrhoea and excretion of oocysts in the
faeces. Oocysts can be detected in faecal smears stained by Giemsa's
method. Infection should be confirmed where possible by histological
demonstration of cryptosporidia attached to the microvillous borders of
ileal enterocytes in recently dead or killed moribund animals.

PATHOLOGY IN LAMBS

In experimental infections of lambs, the small and large intestines
were intensely congested, and mesenteric lymph nodes enlarged and oede-
matous. Cryptosporidia were found throughout both small and large
intestines, different stages of the life-cycle being readily distinguished
in close proximity in the epithelium. The terminal ileum was usually
most severely affected. The main changes were widespread villous atrophy,
with fusion and epithelial cross-bridging between villi. The mucosa was
hyperaemic, and the lamina propria infiltrated by numerous neutrophils.
Cuboidal cells often replaced the more normal columnar enterocytes.

SIGNIFICANCE

The cryptosporidium isolated from calves infected, with or without
causing diarrhoea, a range of domestic and laboratory animals (Tzipori

et al, submitted for publication).   However, the prevalence and hence
the economic importance of cryptosporidiosis is unknown.   We are
currently developing serological tests by which the distribution of the
parasite may be determined.   Recent transmission of human cryptosporidium to animals (Tzipori et al, submitted for publication) suggests
that epidemiological studies may have wider implications in comparative
medicine.

REFERENCES

Levine, N.D.: Protozoan parasites of domestic animals and of man.
    Burgess, Minneapolis, Minnesota (1973).

Pohlenz, J., Bemrick, W.J., Moon, H.W. and Cheville, N.F.: Bovine crypto-
    sporidiosis: a transmission and scanning electron microscopic study
    of some stages in the life cycle and of the host-parasite relation-
    ship.   Vet. Pathol. 15, 417-427 (1978).

Snodgrass, D.R., Angus, K.W., Gray, E.W., Keir, W.A. and Clerihew, L.W.:
    Cryptosporidia associated with rotavirus and an Escherichia coli in an
    outbreak of calf scour.   Vet. Rec. 106, 458-459 (1980).

Tzipori, S., Campbell, I., Sherwood, D., Snodgrass, D.R. and Whitelaw, A.:
    An outbreak of calf diarrhoea attributed to cryptosporidial infection.
    Vet. Rec. in press (1980).

Vetterling, J.M., Jervis, H.R., Merrill, T.G. and Sprinz, H.: Crypto-
    sporidium wrairi sp. n. from the guinea pig cavia porcellus, with an
    emendation of the genus.   J. Protozool. 18, 243-247 (1971).

LIST OF PARTICIPANTS

BELGIUM

Dr. P. DEBOUCK

Faculteit van de Diergeneeskunde
Laboratorium voor Virologie
Casinoplein 24
B - 9000 Gent

Dr. E. van OPDENBOSCH

Nationaal Instituut voor Diergeneeskundig
 Onderzoek
Groeselenberg 99
B - 1180 Brussel (Uccle)

DENMARK

Dr. P.C. GRAUBALLE

Institute of Medical Microbiology
Department of Clinical Virology
University of Copenhagen
22 Juliane Maries Vej
DK - 2100 Copenhagen

FRANCE

Prof. Dr. R. SCHERRER

Station de Recherches de Virologie et
 d'Immunologie (I.N.R.A.)
Route de Thiverval
F - 78850 Thiverval-Grignon

IRELAND

Dr. P. LENNIHAN

Veterinary Research Laboratory
Abbotstown
Castleknock
IRL - County Dublin

ITALY

Prof. Dr. J. Poli

Università di Milano
Via Celoria 10
I - 20133 Milano

THE NETHERLANDS

Dr. D.J. ELLENS
Dr. P.W. de LEEUW

Centraal Diergeneeskundig Instituut
Weverstraat 71
NL - 8223 AB Lelystad

Dr. P.A.M. GUINEE

Rijksinstituut voor de Volksgezondheid
P.O. Box 3
NL - Bilthoven

SWEDEN

Prof. Dr. T. WADSTROM

Dept. of Bacteriology and Epizootiology
Swedish University of Agricultural Sciences
S751
23 Uppsala

UNITED KINGDOM

Visiting Scientists

Dr. J.C. BRIDGER
Dr. R. SELLWOOD

Institute for Research on Animal Diseases
Compton Nr. Newbury
Berks
England

Dr. M.S. McNULTY

Veterinary Research Laboratories
Stormont
Belfast   BT3 3SD
N. Ireland

Dr. S. Tzipori

Animal Diseases Research Association
Moredun Institute
408 Gilmerton Road
Edinburgh   EH17 7JH
Scotland

UNITED STATES OF AMERICA

Dr. C.A. MEBUS

Plum Island Animal Disease Center
P.O. Box 848
Greenport
New York 11944

COMMISSION OF THE EUROPEAN COMMUNITIES (CEC)

Dr. A. PIAVAUX

CEC
VI F 4
200 rue de la Loi
1040 Bruxelles
Belgique